A

NEW PLAN

FOR

SPEEDILY INCREASING

THE

NUMBER OF BEE-HIVES,

&c. &c. &c.

A

NEW PLAN

FOR

SPEEDILY INCREASING

THE

NUMBER OF BEE-HIVES

IN

SCOTLAND;

AND WHICH MAY BE EXTENDED, WITH EQUAL SUCCESS,

TO

ENGLAND, IRELAND, AMERICA,

OR

TO ANY OTHER PART OF THE WORLD CAPABLE OF PRODUCING FLOWERS.

BY JAMES BONNER, BEE-MASTER,

AUTHOR OF PRACTICAL WARPING MADE EASY, &c.

Though small's the Insect, great will be the Gain ;
If heavenly Powers permit, and Phœbus not disdain.

VIRG.

EDINBURGH:

PRINTED BY J. MOIR, PATERSON'S COURT:
SOLD BY W. CREECH, BELL & BRADFUTE, P. HILL, MUDIE & SON,
AND BY THE AUTHOR, AT MR GRANT'S, LEITH WYND,
EDINBURGH :—AND BY T. KAY, NO. 332.
STRAND, LONDON.

1795.

Price 4s. 6d.

MOST NOBLE,

THE PRESIDENT,

AND THE OTHER

RIGHT HONOURABLE

AND HONOURABLE MEMBERS

OF THE

HIGHLAND SOCIETY OF SCOTLAND.

MY LORDS AND GENTLEMEN,

THE generous and diſtinguiſhed mark of reſpect already beſtowed upon me, for my ſmall exertions in the ſervice of the Public, while it commanded my gratitude, at the ſame time emboldened me to ſolicit your Patronage to the following ſheets, wrote upon the important ſubject which firſt introduced me to your notice. Your ready and unanimous acquieſcence, in granting me this additional honour, with the particular favours I have received from many of you, adds exceedingly to the

obligations

obligations formerly beſtowed, and calls for freſh ebullitions of my utmoſt gratitude to you, both as a Society and as Individuals.

THAT your laudable endeavours, for promoting the good of your Country, in every reſpect, may be crowned with the greateſt ſucceſs, and that both the preſent and future generations may be extenſively benefited by your public-ſpirited and patriotic exertions, is the earneſt wiſh of,

MY LORDS AND GENTLEMEN,

Your moſt obedient,

Moſt obliged, and

Moſt humble Servant,

JAMES BONNER.

EDINBURGH,
JULY 18. 1795.

PREFACE.

Biographers and Philosophers are equally puzzled to account for the great diverſity of talents among mankind, and the peculiar bent of genius to be found in each individual. While ſome pretend to account for theſe peculiarities, from the accidental circumſtances in which individuals happen to be placed, others, with at leaſt equal probability, attribute them to peculiar inclinations, implanted by Nature, or rather the Author of Nature in the human mind. Perhaps both cauſes muſt co-operate to produce that degree of enthuſiaſtic fondneſs for particular purſuits, which, in all ages, has diſtinguiſhed ſome individuals in every branch of ſcience, or of art, and which is ſo humorouſly entitled by the facetious STERNE, a man's HOBBY HORSE. *

The author of this work has been, almoſt from his infancy, an admirer of bees, and the

a   fruit

---

* Triſtram Shandy, vol. 1.

fruit of their labours. When a fchool-boy, he read with peculiar pleafure, the defcription given of CANAAN, as a land flowing with milk and HONEY.

Being appointed by his father,* when a boy, to watch his bees in fwarming time, his fondnefs for thefe wonderful infects daily increafed; and he could not help thinking himfelf in a kind of paradifaical ftate, when employed in this delightful office in his father's garden, and running

---

* The author's father, JAMES BONNER, was, like himfelf, fond of rearing bees, and often had a dozen of hives at a time in his garden. He lived above 50 years in the married ftate, and had twelve children, of whom the author is the youngeft alive. He frequently boafted, that, in good feafons, he made as much money by his bees, as nearly purchafed oat-meal fufficient to ferve his numerous family for the whole year. He purchafed a large quarto Bible with the wax produced in one year from his hives, which ferved as a family book ever after; and his houfe was always well fupplied with honey, and a kind of weak mead, which ferved for drink at all feafons of the year. As he lived regularly and temperately, he preferved a great degree of health and vigour to the laft; and was employed in his ordinary bufinefs of weaving, till within a few days of his death; which happened in the 86th year of his age, when he left four fons and a daughter, to regret his lofs. He had always an uncommonly retentive memory; for, upon the fmalleft hint, he could repeat almoft any paffage in fcripture verbatim. He ufed often to entertain his family with a narrative of his treatment of his bees, and of the profit, as well as pleafure, which he had in keeping them.

running among the blooming bushes, and variegated flowers, to look after the young swarms. When very young, he purchased three hives, which he gradually increased to a pretty large stock, and has ever since taken great pleasure, over and above every view of emolument, to study the nature of these valuable insects, and to investigate the causes of their thriving and unprosperous states; their health and diseases; the best means of preserving the individuals, and of propagating and multiplying their industrious race, with their management in every respect. For this purpose, he has perused with avidity every book in the English language, on the subject, that he could get access to; and has spared neither time, trouble, nor expence, (having bestowed much indeed of both, beyond what he could well afford,) in trying numerous experiments upon them.*

a 2   But

* So great was the author's curiosity, and enthusiastic attachment to the study of the nature and properties of these curious insects, that, above twenty years ago, he went from Berwickshire to London, on purpose to converse with Mr WILDMAN on the subject; but that gentleman happening to be in France at the time, he contented himself with purchasing every book he could find on the management of bees, and has ever since made it
his

PREFACE.

But, however valuable and useful many of
the treatises already published·on this subject
have been, he is confident, from the repeated
obfervations and experiments he has made,
that moſt of them are not only defective, but
even erroneous in many particulars; and that
the culture of bees in Britain ‡, has never
yet arrived at any thing near that degree of
perfection, to which it might be brought, if
the ſyſtem which he has formed, and now ſub-
mits to the public, were generally underſtood
and properly practiſed. If we only conſider
the almoſt infinite number of mellifluous flowers, which perfume the air in the honey ſeaſon; and, in particular, the white clover, which
ſo generally and profitably now overſpreads
ſo large a part of our lands in graſs; the various

his chief pleaſure, as well as buſineſs, to ſtudy every poſſible improvement reſpecting that wonderful race. During the honey
ſeaſon, he has often been ſo intent upon this ſtudy, that he hardly allowed himſelf ſleep for whole weeks together.

‡ Although the author, in making out his calculations relative to the increaſe of Bee hives, was under the neceſſity of
confining himſelf to ſome one particular country, and naturally
made choice of his native land, his plan will, nevertheleſs, he
is confident, apply with equal propriety to ENGLAND, IRELAND,
AMERICA, or indeed any other part of the known world, capable
of producing proper food for theſe inſects.

rious fpecies of muftard, and plants of a fimilar kind, found ftill in our corn fields, together with the vaft abundance of heath, that grows fpontaneoufly on our extenfive moors and hills, we may juftly fay, how large and numerous, are our pafture grounds, but how very few are our flocks to feed on them !

A judicious author juftly obferves, that the culture of bees is a branch of rural œconomy, the more valuable, that it is within the reach of the pooreft cottager, and requires neither plowing, manure, cattle, nor rich meadows. All that is wanted, is a fmall degree of attendance, which may be given by the meaneft, as it is requifite only for a fhort time ; and therefore the plentiful harveft of honey and wax that is produced, may be confidered as fo many RICH CROPS REAPED WITHOUT SOWING.

As nothing is fo hurtful to bees as bad weather, fo nothing can be fo little counteracted ; although even the bad effects of it may, in fome meafure, be prevented ; for, we can preferve our bees in cold and fnowy winters, by confining them ; and, in a late fpring, or rainy fummer, we can preferve them from famine, by feeding them properly. But, even in the moft unfavourable weather, I never defpond ; for

I

I have obferved, that in the very worſt feafons, and notwithſtanding the fmall number
of hives, that there are in Scotland, a tolerable quantity of honey is always produced:
And therefore, had there been 20 times more
hives in the kingdom, and a few flowers artificially raiſed, with proper attention, there
would have been, even in theſe very bad feafons, juſt 20 times as much honey and wax
collected as there was: and in good feafons,
fuch as laſt year, (1794) when there was a
great deal of honey produced, even from our
fmall ſtock of hives, what an immenfe quantity would have been collected, had there been
forty or fifty times more ſtock hives in fpring!

Impreffed with thefe ideas, and anxious to
do all in his power to promote an object fo beneficial to the country at large, as well as to
individuals, the author firſt ventured to lay
his fentiments before the public in 1789, by
publiſhing a Treatiſe on the Management of
Bees, which, he was happy to find, attracted
the notice, and procured him the patronage, of
many refpectable and public-fpirited gentlemen. Encouraged by thefe flattering marks
of approbation, he had thoughts of publiſhing a fecond edition; but as, in the continued

nued profecution of this his favourite ftudy, he has made a number of very important difcoveries relative to thefe ufeful infects, he thought it better to prefent thefe new ideas, along with the fubftance of his former work, compreffed into as fmall bounds as poffible, in a new form, and under a new title, than merely to reprint the old work with additions. And the chief object of the prefent performance being to excite the attention of the public in general, but efpecially of gentlemen in opulent circumftances, to the rearing of bees, by fhowing them the PRACTICABILITY of increafing the number of bee-hives in this country at leaft TWENTY-FOLD, if not to FIFTY times the number there are at prefent, he thought it proper to entitle the whole mafs of old and new matter, " A New Plan for fpeedi-" ly increafing the number of Bee-Hives in " Scotland, &c."

Nor is it to his literary labours alone, that he has been indebted for the liberal encouragement he has met with. In his *commercial* concerns, as a dealer in honey, he has been honoured with the patronage and employment of a number of the nobility and gentry in Edinburgh, Newcaftle, and many other places;

for

for which he embraces this opportunity of returning them his beft thanks. And here he
cannot help mentioning a circumftance which
he efteems peculiarly fortunate, as it introduced him to the employment and patronage
of that refpectable patriot, the PRESIDENT OF
THE BOARD OF AGRICULTURE; whofe exer-
ons for the improvement of his country, and
general benefit of fociety, far exceed his praife.
One morning in autumn laft (1794) as the author was carrying a few very fine honey combs,
to a gentleman in the New Town, he was met
by Sir John Sinclair, whom previoufly he did
not know, * and was defired to bring to him
fome of his fine honey next morning. This
he accordingly did, and a converfation having
enfued, refpecting the time he had fpent in
the culture of bees, the number of hives he
kept, &c. &c. he was defired by the public-fpirited Baronet to draw up a plan for the rearing
of bees in a more extenfive manner: and the
author having executed this tafk to the beft of
his

* About a year before this, feveral gentlemen had defired the
author to wait upon Sir JOHN SINCLAIR, and lay before him a
plan for the rearing of bees; but diffidence always prevented him, and probably ever would, if Providence had not brought
about the interview in fome fuch manner as the above-mentioned.

his abilities, Sir John Sinclair was kind enough to lay it before the Highland Society, who were fo good as to honour him with one of their higheft premiums, for his unremitting and fuccefsful attention, during a period of no lefs than 26 years, in acquiring a knowledge of the operations of bees; and for the various difcoveries made by him, tending to multiply the number of hives, and quantity of honey and wax in this kingdom, contained in his communications to the fociety, and now laid before the public, in this treatife.

This encouragement led the author to hope, that his plan might turn out to be generally a-dopted, if once univerfally known. He there-fore diftributed fubfcription papers, in order to try the minds of the public in general; and in doing this, his fuccefs far exceeded his moft fanguine expectations; for he fcarcely met with one in an hundred, who did not ap-prove of his plan; as will appear from the refpectable lift of fubfcriptions prefixed to this work, and which might have been rendered greatly more numerous, if the author's time and other avocations had permitted him to circulate his propofals more generally.

b   The

The author, therefore, without farther apology, now submits his plan to the attention of the public; and he has not a doubt, but that, if the directions therein given are strictly adhered to, and persevered in by gentlemen of property, and the public in general, in a few years Scotland will not only save much money now sent abroad for honey and wax, but will even be able to render them articles of export.

He needs only add, that, in the following treatise, he has not, as too many authors in all branches of science are apt to do, strained any arguments to support a favourite hypothesis: But, on the contrary, his whole theory and practice being founded on experience and facts, he flatters himself, that he has delivered his sentiments throughout the work, in a manner so plain and intelligible, that the most unlettered reader will not mistake his meaning.

NAMES OF THE SUBSCRIBERS.

A

Jacob Atkinson, Esq; Newcastle

Reverend Mr Allison, Newburn

Mr James Arbuthnot, jun. Peterhead,

Messrs Allan and West, booksellers, No. 15, Paternoster-row, London, 12 copies

Mr Alexander Aitchison, student of physic, Edinburgh

B.

Colonel Baillie, of Rosehall, 2 copies

Reverend Doctor George Baird, principal of the University of Edinburgh

John Balfour, Esq; of Balbirnie

A. Barclay, Esq; W. S. Edinburgh

John Bell, Esq; of Gallow-hill 2 copies

Benjamin Bell, Esq; surgeon, Edinburgh

Andrew Bell, Esq; engraver, Edinburgh

William Beveridge, Esq; W. S. Edin.

David Black, Esq; Dunfermline

John Bogue, Esq; of Halydown

William Bogue, Esq; of Greenburn

Thomson Bonnar, Esq; Edinburgh

Alexander Boswell, Esq; of Auchenleck

George Brown, Esq; one of the Commissioners of Excise, Edinburgh

Thomas Bruce, Esq; of Arnot, 2 copies

Thomas Bruce, Esq; of Kennet

Edward Bruce, Esq; W. S. Edinburgh

Arthur Bruce, Esq; Secretary to the Natural History Society, Edinburgh

John Buchan, Esq; W. S. Edinburgh

Mr John Buchan, accountant, Edinburgh

Hector M'Donald Buchanan, Esq; W. S. Edinburgh

John Butter, Esq; of Benbecula

Captain Abraham Bunbury

Reverend Mr George Bowe, Shilbottle

Reverend Mr John Brodie, Kinloch

Reverend Mr Laurence Butler, Lethendy

Messrs Bell and Bradfute, booksellers, Edinburgh, 6 copies

Messrs Beilby and Bewick, Newcastle.

Mrs Baker, Edinburgh

John Barclay, A. M. Edinburgh

Mr Peter Bathgate, weaver, Ayton

Mr Robert Baillie

Mr Robert Bowmaker, Chirnside

Mr Robert Brown, coal owner, Wickham

Mr Michael Brown, Morpeth

Mr John Bonner, Stitchel (copies

Mr David Bonner, Woolwich, 2:0.

Mrs Beatrix Bonner, Auchencrow

C

Hon. John Campbell, Lord Stonefield, 2 copies

Alexander Christie, Esq; of Gruel-dykes, sheriff depute, Berwick-shire

Duncan Campbell, Esq; sheriff substitute of Argyllshire

David Campbell, Esq; of Combie

John Campbell, Esq; of Auch

Ewen Cameron, Esq; of Falsfern

William Cadell, Esq; of Banton

George Cadell, Esq; Edinburgh

James Carfrae, Esq; merchant, Edinburgh

James

James Clark, M. D. Newcastle

Thomas Cleghorn, Efq; coachmaker, Edinburgh

B. Clifton, Efq; Edinburgh

T. S. Conftantius, Efq;

Andrew Coventry, M. D. Profeffor of Agriculture, Edinburgh, 3 copies

William Creech, Efq; bookfeller, Edinburgh 24 copies

Thomas Curtis, Efq; Edinburgh

Captain John Cowe, Edinburgh

Reverend Mr Chalmers, Haddington

Reverend Mr William Chalmers, Auchtergaven

Mr Robert Campbell, fherriff clerk, Invernefs, 2 copies

Mr George Charlton, Newcaftle

Mr William Charnley, bookfeller, Newcaftle

Mr William Crawford, Edinburgh

Mr Robert Currie, apothecary, Newcaftle

D

Dowager Lady Dundas, of Kerfe, 2 copies

George Dempfter, Efq; of Dunnichen, 3 copies (copies

William Darnell, Efq; Newcaftle, 2

Reverend Thomas Davidfon, of Muirhoufe, D. D.

William Dawfon, Efq; Frogton 4 cop.

Captain Deans, of the Royal Navy, Huntington

James Donaldfon, Efq; printer, Edin.

Colin Drummond, M. D. Edinburgh

James Drummond, Efq; of Strageath

Keith Dunbar, Efq; Edinburgh

John Dyfon, Efq; glafs manufacturer, Newcaftle

Mrs Dirom, Queen Street, Edinburgh

Mrs C. Durham, George's Square, Edinburgh

Mr John Dennis, Newcaftle

Mr Thomas Dixon, Glafs-houfe, Newcaftle

Mr James Donaldfon, Dundee

Mr John Doxford, Morpeth

E

Thomas Elder Efq; of Forneth, Poftmafter General, and late Lord Provoft of Edinburgh

James Elliot, Efq; Queen Street, Edinburgh (3 copies

James Francis Erfkine, Efq; of Marr,

Reverend John Erfkine of Carnock, D. D. Edinburgh (pies

James Erfkine, Efq; of Cardrofs 2 copies

Methven Erfkine, Efq; of Cambo

Mr James Elder, fadler, Edinburgh

F

Honourable Archibald Frafer of Lovat, 5 copies

Colonel Ferrier, Edinburgh, Scotch Brigades

George Fairbolme, Efq; of Greenknow.

Francis Farquharfon, Efq; of Oughton

William Fife, Efq; furgeon, Newcaftle

Captain John Forbes, royal navy

James Forman, Efq; W. S. Edinburgh (copies

Jofeph Forfter, Efq; of Setonburn 2

—— Forfter, M. D. Newtown of the Sea, Northumberland

James Frafer, Efq; of Gortuleg, W. S. Edinburgh

William Fullarton, Efq; (copies

Mr Thomas Fair, tenant, Refton, 2

Mr John Fellfhaw, of Southwell

Mr Fletcher, gardener, Reftalrig

G

Sir John Gordon of Invergordon. Bart.

Thomas

Thomas Gillespie, M. D. Edinburgh
Lewis Gordon, Esq; Depute Secretary of the Highland Society, Edin.
James Farquhar Gordon, Esq; Edinburgh
——Gordon, Esq; W. S. Edinburgh
——Gordon, Esq; Edinburgh
James Grant, Esq; of Corriemony, advocate
John Gray, Esq; W. S. Edinburgh
Reverend William Greenfield, D. D. Professor of Rhetoric, Edinburgh
James Grierson, Esq; of Dalgonerie 3 copies
George Grieve, M. D. Newcastle
Reverend Mr William Greig, Longside, Aberdeenshire
Mr Ebenezer Gairdner, merchant, Edinburgh
Mr Benjamin Gibson, Newcastle
Mr John Goldie, gardener
Mr Gordon, vintner, Press Inn
Mr William Grant, weaver's wright, Edinburgh
Mr Alexander Greenfield, portioner, Auchencrow

H

                        (copies
Sir James Hall of Dunglass, Bart. 3
Patrick Home, Esq; of Wedderburn, M. P. Berwickshire, 3 copies
William Hall, Esq; of Whitehall, 3 copies
Alexander Hamilton, M. D. Professor of Midwifery, Edinburgh
James Hamilton, M. D. Edinburgh 2 copies
James Hare, Esq;
Charles Hay, Esq; of Faichfield, advocate   (copies
Robert Hay, Esq; of Drummelzier 10
James Horne, Esq; W. S. Edinburgh, 2 copies
George Home, Esq; of Branxton 4 copies
James Home, Esq; of Fairlaw
P. Hunter, Esq; junior, of Thurston
James Huntly, Esq; surgeon, Gateshead, Newcastle.

Thomas Hutchison, Esq; merchant, Edinburgh
Mr Alexander Hutchison, merchant, Edinburgh
Rev, Mr William Haigh, Newcastle
Mr William Hall, Newcastle
Mr Robert Hay, wright, Edinburgh
Mr Thomas Henderson, Leith
Mr Peter Hill, bookseller, Edinburgh 6 copies
Mr John Hogg, merchant, Newcastle

I

Patrick Inglis, Esq; merchant, Edinburgh
—— Ingrame, M. D. Newcastle
John Innes, Esq; W. S. Edinburgh
Mr William Ingledew, Newcastle

J.

James Jackson, Esq; merchant, Edinburgh
John Jamieson, junior, Esq; Leith
—— Johnston, M. D. Dunbar
Reverend Mr J. Johnston, Alnwick
Mr William Johnston, Factor, Foulden
Mr Johnston, weaver, Newtown of the Muir

K

William Keith, Esq; accomptant, Edinburgh
—— Kentish, Esq; surgeon, Newcastle
Mr Thomas Kay, bookseller, Strand, London, 50 copies

L

William Leavis, Esq; Newcastle
Edward Lothian, Esq; W. S. Edinburgh
Alexander Low, Esq; of Cash

                        Archibald

Jonathan Anderson Ludford, M. D. Clarendon, Jamaica

Archibald Lundie, Efq; W. S. Edin.

Reverend Mr Henry Lundie, Edin.

Reverend Mr James Landels, Coldingham

Mr Herman Lyon, apothecary, Edinburgh

Mr George Lothian, merchant, Glafgow

Mr William Lothian, merchant, Edinburgh

Mr Addifon Langhorn, Newcaftle

Mr M. Lofthoufe, Gatefhead, Newcaftle

Mr John Law, meffenger, Edinburgh

M

Right Honourable Robert M'Queen of Braxfield, Lord Juftice Clerk

Sir Alexander M'Kenzie, of Coull, Baronet, 2 copies

Alexander Monro, M. D. profeffor of anatomy, Edinburgh

Mrs M'Donald of Sanda

Mrs M'Donald, of Clanronald, 2 cop.

Donald M'Donald, Efq; of Kinlochmoidart

Angus M'Donell, Efq; of Auchtrichen

Donald M'Intofh, Efq; writer, Edinburgh

John M'Kenzie, Efq; W. S. Edinburgh

Captain M'Kenzie, Royal Navy

Alexander M'Kenzie, Efq; writer, Edinburgh

William M'Leod, Efq; of Kaimes, fheriff depute of Bute

John M'Murdoch, Efq; Drumlanrick

Lauchlan M'Tavifh, Efq; W. S.

E. Marjoribanks, Efq; Prince's Street, Edinburgh

David Martin, Efq; limner, Edinburgh

Gilbert Meafon, Efq; of Mordun

George Midford, Efq; Morpeth

Archibald Milne, Efq; W. S. Edinburgh, 2 copies

William Molle, Efq; W. S. Ediburgh

Robert Moore, Efq; of Blairtown, Ayrfhire, 2 copies

John Morthland, Efq; advocate, Edin.

James Wolfe Murray, Efq; advocate, Edinburgh

Reverend Mr William M'Ritchie, Clunie

Reverend Mr Robert Mudie, Clackmanan

Mr John Mackie, of Rora

Mr George Mowey, Newcaftle

Mrs Maitland, Gayfield, Edinburgh

Mr Robert M'Kay, manufacturer, Berwick

Archibald M'Kinlay, Efq; merchant, Edinburgh

Mr Daniel M'Queen, Sun-Fire-office, Edinburgh

Mr Hugh M'Whirter, Bleacher, Inglefgreen (copies

Mr George Mickle, Swinton Houfe, 2

Mr Moore, fchoolmafter, Morpeth, 6 copies

Mr Motlay, Morpeth

Meffrs George Mudie and Son, bookfellers, Edinburgh, 12 copies

Mr Andrew Muirhead, Edinburgh

Mr John Moir, printer, Edinburgh, 2 copies

N

John New, Efq;

William Newton, Efq; of Newton

Jofeph Norris, Efq; one of the clerks of Jufticiary, Edinburgh

Mr James Normand, Edinburgh

O

John Ogilvy, Efq; of Gardoch,

Stephen

P

Stephen Pemberton, M. D. Newcastle
Reverend Mr James Playfair, Bendochy
Mr Samuel Paterson, merchant, Edinburgh
Mr James Pentland, merchant, Newcastle
Mr John Proctor, surgeon, Newcastle
Mr Peter Pae, merchant, Coldingham
Mr George Purves, Auchencrow

R

The Hon. David Rae, Lord Eskgrove
Sir Alexander Ramsay Irvine, of Balmain, Baronet
Peter Ramsay, Esq; younger of Barnton, banker, Edinburgh
J Ramsay, M. D. Newcastle, 2 cop.
David Ramsay, Esq; printer, Edinburgh
George Rennie, Esq; Linton (copies
Alexander Renton, Esq; Lamberton, 6
John Robertson, Esq; Lauriston (burgh
Adam Rolland, Esq; advocate, Edin-
Adam Rolland, Esq; W. S. Edinburgh
Colin Ross, Esq; of Castlemilk
Matthew Ross, Esq; advocate, Edin.
Walter Ross, Esq; factor on the estate of Cromarty, 2 copies
—— Ross, Esq; of Kilmanivaig 2
Reverend Mr John Robertson, Little Dunkeld
—— Redpath, M. D. Berwick, 2 cop.
Mr Charles Raitt, woad manufacturer, Newcastle
—— Reid, Esq; builder, Edinburgh
Mr Thomas Robson, sadler, Morpeth
Mr Robson, ship-builder, Newcastle
Mr Thomas Robson, wharfinger, Newcastle

S

Right Hon. Sir James Stirling, Bart. Lord Provost of Edinburgh (copies
Hon. David Smith, Lord Methven 2

Hon. John Swinton, Lord Swinton
Hon. Sir John Sinclair, of Ulbster Bart. M. P. President of the Board of Agriculture, &c. 7 copies
Hon. Lady Diana Sinclair, of Ulbster
Hon. Lady Janet Sinclair, of Ulbster
P. Sandilands, Esq; Edinburgh
Dominico Felix Dos Santos, M. D. Brazil (copies
William Scott, Esq; of Friershaw, 3
George Shadforth, Esq; Newcastle
George Sinclair, Esq; merchant, Leith
Joseph Smith, Esq; Meadow-house 2 copies
—— Sommerville, Esq; surgeon, Haddington 3 copies (burgh
Andrew Stewart, Esq; W. S. Edinburgh
Charles Stewart, M. D. Edinburgh
Francis Strachan, Esq; W. S. Edinburgh
James Strachan, Esq; W. S. Edinburgh
Nathan Surgeon, Esq; surgeon, Newcastle
Reverend Mr Sharp, Coldingham
Reverend Mr Shepherd, Bolam
Reverend Mr William Syme, Newcastle
Mr Alexander Scott, Coldingham
Messrs Thomas and William Sommers, vintners, Edinburgh
Mr Alexander Steel, merchant, Edinburgh
Mr Strange, teacher of dancing, Edinburgh
Mr Robert Swanston, tenant, Newfarm

T

John Tawze, Esq; W. S. Edinburgh
Anthony Taylor, Esq; Infirmary, Newcastle
J Thompson, M. D. Gayfield, Edinburgh
Charles Thomson, Esq; Edinburgh
Thomas Tod, Esq; Edinburgh
Thomas Tod, junior, Esq; George's Square, Edinburgh

Alexander

Alexander Tweedie, Esq; of Quarter
John Tweedie, Esq; writer, Edinburgh
Mr Robert Tweedie, merchant, Edinburgh
Reverend Mr Robert Trotter, Morpeth
Mr John Tajt, joiner, Guyzon
Mr Thomas Taylor, Newburn
Mr Robert Thomson, merchant, Edinburgh
Mr Andrew Thompson, Lauder
Mr Thomas Thompson, inn-keeper, Gateside
Mr William Thomson, Haddington
Mr James Thorburn, grocer, Edinburgh
Mr Train, engraver, Bourdeau house

U

James Ure, Esq; Comptroller of the Customs, Alloa
Reverend David Ure, A. M. Edinburgh

V

Caspar Voght, Esq; Hamburgh
John Veitch, Esq; Surgeon, Ayton

W

Andrew Wardrop, Esq; surgeon, Edinburgh
John Wilson, Esq; Morpeth
James Wood, M. D. Newcastle
Mrs Alexander Wood, Edinburgh
George Wood, Esq; surgeon, Edinburgh
Reverend Mr Wilson, Ayton
Mr James Watson, merchant, Newcastle
Mr Walker, North America
Mrs Wardlaw, Edinburgh
Mrs Watson, Charlotte Square, Edin.
Mr William Watson, upholsterer, Edinburgh
Mr John White, schoolmaster, Ayton
Mr Robert Whitfield, Morpeth
Mr Joseph Whitfield, bookseller, Newcastle
Mr George Whitlaw, Ayton
Mr ———— Woodman, Morpeth

Y

Mr Ebenezer Young, bailie of Dunse
Mr John Young, Edinburgh

A considerable number of subscriptions, besides those above inserted, have been obtained for this work, which the author is sorry he cannot insert, his correspondents not having yet transmitted him their lists.

CONTENTS

CONTENTS.

CHAP.

NEW

NEW PLAN

FOR

SPEEDILY INCREASING

THE

NUMBER OF BEE-HIVES

IN

SCOTLAND.

CHAP. I.

OF THE PLEASURE AND PROFIT, THAT ATTEND THE KEEPING OF BEES.

BEES, thofe emblems of virtue, have long been the ftudy and delight of wife men, and have employed the ableft pens in many nations, and in different ages. In the facred writings, the land of Canaan is fpoken of as a good land, and, as an evidence of its being fo, it is called a land flowing with milk and *honey*. Among the ancients, Ariftomachus contemplated bees for the fpace of fifty-eight

A   years;

years ; and Philiſcus retired into the woods,
that he might have more convenient opportunities of obſerving them. Among the moderns, I ſhall juſt only mention Purchas, Rouſ-
den, Geddie, Butler, Warder, Bradley, Thorly,
Thomas and Daniel Wildman, Stephen and
William White, and Keys, all Engliſhmen,
and Robert Maxwell, a Scotchman ;—all of
whom have publiſhed treatiſes on them, the
moſt of which have appeared within this
century; and they have given many uſeful directions how to manage bees, according to the
knowledge they had attained to, reſpecting
that admirable inſect.

The knowledge of bees, like that of many
other things, is found out by degrees, and may
be ſaid, in ſome meaſure, to be ſtill but in a ſtate
of infancy, as appears by the many miſtakes fal-
len into, and taught by thoſe who have wrote
on that ſubject, notwithſtanding their fair pro-
miſes in their title pages ; as—" A Complete
" Guide for the management of Bees," &c. They
have all been ſtrangely miſled in their opinion
about the generation of bees, aſſerting that the
Queen lays three different kind of eggs, *viz.*
one kind for the production of the Queen Bee,
another for that of the Working Bees, and a
third

third for the Drones; an opinion, which the author of the following sheets will, he humbly hopes, prove to be erroneous.

As in every undertaking there is some leading motive, which excites us to engage in it, so the rearing of bees is attended with a degree both of profit and pleasure, highly deserving the attention of the philosopher, the gentleman-farmer, and the industrious peasant. What is more pleasant, than to observe the labours of a hive of bees in the spring, when the days begin to lengthen, and frost and snow, like birds of darkness, cannot bear the sun! Then these industrious creatures begin to fly about, and dance and sing, rejoicing at the return of the genial season! Then they reform what is amiss in the hive, and, as their family enlarges, they omit no opportunity of gathering in fresh provision for their increasing young. In the honey season, how delightful to see them hurrying in their yellow loads! How diligent they are to lay up provision for the returning winter! View them in this smiling clover field, or yonder flowery mead! See how busily they work! And hear how sweetly they sing! How pleasant to behold a swarm of bees lightly flying in the air, and darkening the heavens

A 2   with

with a thoufand varying lines ! Now, behold the innumerable tribe, formed into one compact body, fufpended from yonder verdant fhrub, eftablifhing themfelves into an independent colony, while their careful mafter, with confcious delight, meditates on his increafing ftore!

Bees, when properly managed, are alfo very profitable, as, in good years, moft hives will throw two fwarms; in moderate years, one. Although, in bad years, perhaps, fome will fwarm none at all, yet, eftimating by moderate years, and allowing each hive, one with another, to fwarm only once, which valuing at 15s. each, twenty ftock hives will thereby yield their mafter 15l. yearly;—no fmall fum to be got with fo much pleafure, and fo little toil. They will yield that much, although one or two fhould die in winter; nor need any think my eftimate too high; if their hives be good, they will have that much one year with another. For example, in fummer 1787, the advantage arifing from bees was fuch, that many proprietors of them made 30s. and fome even 40s. of one fingle hive; and in March 1788, I fold a hive to a neighbour of mine, which in the following fummer

mer increased to five, four of which he set aside for stock hives that autumn.

As there is no concern, in rural œconomy, more profitable than bees, in favourable seasons, considering the trifling expence that attends them, we shall here give an estimate to what extent bees may be reared, and also what their value may amount to in ten years.

Suppose, for instance, one should begin with five hives, which will cost him 5l., no great sum to commence bee-master with, and allowing each hive, one with another, to double their number, they will increase in the following proportions:

Years.	Hives.
1	5
2	10
3	20
4	40
5	80
6	160
7	320
8	640
9	1280
10	2560

Thus,

Thus, in the fpace of 10 years, 5 hives will produce 2560 fwarms, which, valued at 10s. each hive, a very moderate eftimation, amounts to 1280l. clear profit; allowing the fecond and third fwarm to pay for hives, ftools, labour, and incidental loffes.

By the above calculation, my reader muft not conclude, that every hive of bees will produce fo many; but, I confidently affert, that many have done fo, and much more, in proportion, according to the time they have ftood; but, fuppofing 160 of thefe hives fhould fail by cold, robbers, famine, or bad management, during the above mentioned years, there will ftill remain 1200l. of clear profit.

Let it alfo be confidered here, that by the above eftimation, it is taken for granted, that the feafons are very favourable for bees, being fine, calm, funny warm weather, with foft fhowers now and then, and alfo plenty of good pafture in their neighbourhood, whereon they will work and fing without moleftation; wantonly fkipping from flower to flower, and rifling all their fweets, rejoicing that they are amply provided with fuch plenty of provifion, while the fmiling fun invites them to enjoy it. With what delight have I often witneffed my

induftrious

induftrious fervants carrying on their work
with fo much fimplicity, alacrity, and chearfulnefs, and finging fo fweetly ; infomuch that
they are fit to make me join the concert, and
fing,

What's this I hear, makes fuch melodious found !
Surely I've got on fome enchanted ground.
'Tis Canaan's infects that I here behold,
Whofe legs do glitter like the yellow gold.
The furze and broom in luftre here do fhine,
Whofe yellow tops regale thofe flocks of mine.
Here filver ftreams in flow'ry valleys glide,
And rows of willows deck the river's fide :
Here lambkins play upon the funny braes,
And fweeteft nectar fmells on clover lees.
Here are the fields with Nature's colours dight,
Grateful to fmell, and pleafant to the fight.
Retired pleafure foothes and calms the mind ;
A noify world oft leaves a fting *behind.*

On the contrary, however, fhould the feafon
go to the other extreme, and, inftead of fair weather, fhould windy, cold, wet, cloudy, and heavy
weather take place, during fummer, the bees
will by it be fo much difheartened and difcouraged, that they will lament and mourn, in fo
piteous

piteous and difconfolate a manner, that they have
often made fuch an impreffion on my fpirits,
that I was fit to mourn along with them.   The
truth is, I have often thought that there was
fomething of the nature of a bee in myfelf; as
always when they are happy, and rejoicing, fo
am I; when they are mourning and difconfolate, my fpirits are alfo low; when fighting
and plundering from one another, my temper
is fo chagrined, that it is with difficulty I re-
ftrain the effects of my ill humour; infomuch,
that my domeftics, with little knowledge in
phyfiognomy, can eafily judge from the chearfulnefs, depreffion, or chagrin, apparent on my
countenance, the ftate and temper of my little
republics.*

It

* A two-fold reafon may be affigned for this. Fine weather
enlivens the animal fpirits, whereas a dull fky, and a cloudy atmof-
phere, generally produce the contrary effect.   In the latter
cafe, the bees can do nothing but confume a part of that delicious
ftore, which they had laid up for their own and their mafter's ufe.
Sympathy and intereft are therefore equally excited, by fuch
weather, to produce this effect; and ftill more by the circumftance
of their killing one another; for that man muft be callous, indeed,
to every feeling of humanity, who can, with indifference, behold
numbers of fuch ufeful and induftrious animals, lying like fo many
murdered heroes on the field of battle, mutually flain by each o-
ther; not to add, that a perfon of the moft ftoical difpofition muft
feel fomewhat ruffled, at the lofs of fo many ufeful fervants,
whom he would do every thing in his power to preferve.

In fuch unfavourable feafons, bees increafe fo very little, that, perhaps, the owner can fcarcely collect, from among all his hives, as many good ones, as will keep up his ftock properly for the next feafon; but as fuch bad feafons does not happen often, it fhould not difcourage any perfon from commencing beemafter, as even, in the very worft, with proper care, the ftock may always be preferved, which is not the cafe with many other articles in which mankind deal.

It is hardly neceffary to obferve, that bees have amazingly thriven laft year, as almoft every hive produced twice, and many even thrice; and confequently, the price of honey has thereby been greatly reduced, from what it was in former years.

CHAP. II.

OF THE APIARY.

As a general rule, place your hives where they will be leaft expofed to the wind, and enjoy as much of the influence of the fun as poffible; for wind always retards the bees in their work,

B   while

while the fun's beams invite them to it. Although it is well known, that bees will thrive well in high and windy fituations, yet a low one is always to be preferred. In the neighbourhood of the apiary, there fhould be abundance of flowers, from which the bees may collect their wax and honey.

Were a choice allowed me, where to place my bees, it would be in an early fituation,—a hollow glen by the fide of a rivulet, furrounded with abundance of turnips in bloffom, in the fpring,—muftard and clover in fummer,—and heath in the latter end of fummer and harveft ; with a variety of other garden and wild flowers in their feafons. However I would not be underftood, as if I hinted that bees would not thrive, unlefs they were placed in fuch an advantageous fituation, as the contrary can be proved : for bees have thriven amazingly well, in places where they were not within reach of many of the above mentioned flowers ; but although they will do well in moft fituations, and fly far for food, yet they will thrive far better, when fituated among or near good pafture ; and furrounded with abundance of food. This leads us forward to fhew what is the proper pafture for bees, which fhall be the fubject of the following chapter,

G H A P,

CHAP. III.

AMONG the great variety of flowers, which wife Nature has fo profufely laid before our noble infects, from which they may abundantly fupply themfelves with food, we fhall, in the firft place, give fome particular account of thofe five principal ones in this country, from which bees extract vaft quantities of honey;—viz. turnips, rape, muftard, clover and heath; and then conclude this chapter, with fome account of many other excellent flowers which bees feed on.

Turnips, in particular, blow early in the fpring, and continue long in flower; and they alfo yield both honey and farina, by which the bees are greatly excited to go abroad, and work upon them, when perhaps, in late fituations, they have fcarcely any other flower to

B 2   work

work upon. In such places, therefore, it is
highly proper, that turnips be sowed, and allowed to remain in the ground during winter.
Thefe, yielding their flowers from the middle
of March to the end of April, will afford the
bees fix weeks good pasture, and thus render
them equal to thofe in more favourable or earlier fituations ; whereas they would perhaps have
scarcely had any other flower to work upon, that
could do them much good. I would therefore, ftrongly recommend to all proprietors
of bees, particularly thofe in late fituations, if
they can by any means, to let always as
many turnips run into bloffom in the fpring, as
may be fufficient to afford plenty of early pasture
for their bees to work on. Thus the rich may
fupply themfelves with that feed for fowing, and
the poor will have it to fell to thofe who need
it, which will enable them to pay the rent of
the ground they grow upon. But here it may
naturally be afked, By what rule are we to
judge, what quantity of ground will yield a
fufficiency of food for any given number of
hives? I anfwer, that very little ground will
keep many hives abundantly at work; as, for
example, one acre of good land would not be
overftocked with 20 hives; and confequently,
the

the twentieth part of an acre would keep one
in constant employment.

The rape in blossom answers the same end to
bees as the turnips; and as it is a little later of
flowering, it will yield the bees a fresh and
seasonable supply, when the turnips begin to
fade, and thereby keep them constantly at
work till the latter end of May, * when all
the herbs of nature will, as it were, vie with
each other who shall contribute most to supply this noble and virtuous race, with abundance of the sweetest nectar. Then, at this
season, the balmy plane-tree regales them in
the morning, before the drowsy herd ascends
the hill to relieve his imprisoned bleaters: and
the gold-like furze, mustard, and broom, invite them to feast till the day decline.

Garden and wild mustard, with runches of all
kinds, bees are very fond of, and work keenly
thereon; and these flowers are attended with this
advantage, that by sowing their seeds at different times in the Spring, their flowering
may

* The two flowers above mentioned, as they are easily raised,
should be paid particular attention to, in the Highlands of Scotland, or any other Moorland situations, where there are very few
natural flowers growing, except the heath.

may be fo protracted, as to afford the bees a
fufficiency of pafture during the whole working feafon.

In June comes the white clover, which continues long in bloffom, and alfo yields abundance of the fineft of honey: And wherever
the proprietor of bees has it in his power, he
fhould be particularly attentive to raife it in
his pafture lands; and, as I hinted with refpect
to turnips and rape, the clover grafs will
pay the rent of the ground, exclufive of what
advantage the bees derive from it. So fond
are the bees of this flower, that whenever it
appears, they will defert and overlook many
other excellent flowers, as unworthy of their
attention, and eagerly dart upon it, and work
and fing thereon all the day long, until the
cold evening chafe them with reluctance home
to reft: But, as all nature's beauties fade, and
thereby give way to their fucceffors, fo does
this beloved herb, as, about the end of July,
they begin to blacken, and the balmy dew to
forfake their fweeteft lips; then our heroes go
in fearch of frefh provifions, and in their ram-
bles, as they fkim over our lofty mountains,
are attracted by the blue heather bells, which
are numberlefs as the fands on the fea fhore;
each

each one of which, by the affiftance of Phœbus, difclofes its fweets, and thereby invites
the tranfported bee to rifle all their charms.

Heath is attended with this advantage,
that it needs no culture nor rearing; but, on
the contrary, grows fpontaneoufly, in too great
abundance, in many places; as, moft certainly,
the greater half of Britain is covered with it;
but, like the clover, it yields alfo vaft quantities of the fineft honey; and, when the month
of Auguft is favourable warm weather, no
thriving hives of bees, placed near it, need
fail, in a fhort time, to enrich themfelves with
plenty of honey.

The flowers of furze, broom, and plane tree,
as formerly hinted, are highly grateful to bees,
as all of them afford abundance of matter to
collect their honey and wax from. Furze, in
particular, generally flowers early, and continues long in bloffom.

Befides the flowers above mentioned, there
is a great variety of others, which, in their different feafons, afford employment and materials for the bees; fuch as lillies, rofe-marys, yellow
gowans, and the bloffoms of crocufes, fnow-
drops, oziers, fallows, vetches, alders, poppies,
beans, goofeberry bufhes, and fruit trees of all
kinds,

kinds. In fhort, I know no flower that they
will refufe, when they are at a lofs for variety;
for, like the poor among mankind, when a
choice is denied them, they will be contented
with coarfe fare; but give them their option
amongft a variety, and it will foon be perceived,
how little they value the gaudy *fhow*, when put
in competition with *fubftance*; for they will fly
over the fineft gardens, and the moft beautiful
flowers, and cheerfully feed on their beloved
turnips, runches, clover, and heath.

There is one thing very obfervable, that
whatever flower a bee firft pitches upon, fhe
always continues to work upon the fame fpecies, till fhe is loaded, although fhe fhould be
obliged to fly over better kinds, and even to
fome confiderable diftance for them; but, if
the bees cannot obtain a full loading from thofe
flowers which they prefer, they fometimes
make up the remainder from other flowers.

What the honey dew confifts of, is difputed
among the learned. According to the ancients,
it was an efflux of air, a dew which fell upon
flowers. The moderns fay, it is rather a per-
fpiration of the fineft particles of the fap in
plants,

plants, which, evaporating through the pores, afterwards condense upon the flowers *.

" The honey dew (says Mr Key) is not a
" liquid deposited by the air on the leaves of
" plants, as is generally supposed; for then,
" like other dews or fogs, it would fall on,
" and adhere to, all sorts of plants indiscrimi-
" nately; whereas, it is found only on a *few*
" particular plants; and on them but partial-
" ly, for the young leaves afford none.

" This substance is as transparent and as
" sweet as honey, and is, in fact, perfect ho-
" ney, attracted through the pores of the
" leaves, by a peculiar sultry heat; particular-
" ly when reflected through clouds. Some-
" times it is found on the leaves in the form
" of little drops or globules. But, at other
" times, being more diluted by the greater
" moisture of the atmosphere, it covers the
" leaves, as though they were spread with a
" fine syrup.

" The time, in which these honey dews are
" generally found, is from the beginning of
" June to the middle of July. But it will
" vary, in proportion as the weather is wet or

C   " dry;

* Nature Delineated.

" dry; which will occasion them to be either
" sooner or later. The hotteft and drieft fum-
" mers produce the largeft and moft frequent
" honey dews. In cold and wet feafons, few
" or none of them are to be feen.

" Whenever a honey dew is found, the bees
" are fo extremely eager to fetch it, that they
" quit all other work, that their returns may be
" the quicker and more numerous; and left a
" gloomy change fhould deprive them of the
" precious prize. No harveft fwain, dreading
" impending ftorms, can be more anxious or
" expeditious, in haftening the houfing of his
" crops, than thefe aerial tribes in this their
" delightful office; fo much fo, that thronging
" in too great numbers at the door, they
" joftle and tumble each other down. And
" fmarting woe to thofe who fhall thoughtlefs-
" ly ftand in their way at this important cri-
" fis! Their joy on thefe occafions, is ex-
" preffed in fuch inceffant and loud notes, as
" to be heard at a great diftance. By thefe to-
" kens it may be known, that there is a honey
" dew, without feeing the trees from which
" they gather it."

A friend informed me, that he has often
difcovered both bees and ants upon the oak
                                        leaves

leaves, fipping the honey dew; which agrees
nearly with the Abbe BOISSIER DE SAU-
VAGES's account of it, in France, as quoted
by WILDMAN, p. 80, et feq. For my part,
although I have often travelled many miles, in
the fineft weather, to places where oaks were
growing in great abundance, in order to fatisfy myfelf on that point, yet I never could
difcover a fingle drop of honey dew on them,
or any bees to collect it. And many perfons
have affured me, that they never faw a fingle
bee upon an oaken leaf collecting honey. I
am, neverthelefs, far from difcrediting the report; as thofe who are fituated nearer extenfive woods, have doubtlefs much better opportunities of afcertaining this fact, than I. And
that there are honey dews to be difcovered in
fuch fituations, I readily believe; as I have often obferved my own bees collecting honey
from the *outfides* of the fockets of different
flowers, particularly from thofe of the wild
runches, inftead of extracting it by their probofcis from the *infide.* I have fometimes,
though very feldom, obferved them, in a fine
morning, about fun-rife, bufily employed upon
the leaves of the white thorn, at a feafon
when there was not a fingle flower to be feen

on

on it ; which inclines me to think it is not an
efflux of air, as some suppose, but rather a per-
spiration of some of the finest particles of the
sap of plants, which, evaporating through the
pores, afterwards condenses upon the leaves.
At such favourable opportunities, the bees will
doubtless soon fill their hives with honey ;
but I am of opinion, that such happy seasons
are generally very short, and that for many
years they last but a very few days ; and in
some cold years, perhaps they scarcely occur at
all.

Some writers believe, that when the liquor
which the bees collect, has been for some time
in their stomachs, it comes from thence changed into true honey ; the liquor having been
there properly digested, and rendered thicker
than when it entered. Others are of opinion,
that the bee makes no alteration in the honey,
but collects this delicious syrup just as nature
produces it, and first fills her bag, and then
discharges it into the magazine ; which appears to me to be the most probable opinion ;
as I have sometimes taken a bee from a flower
the moment she was collecting the honey, and
torn her asunder, (although with the greatest
reluctance,)

reluctance,) to fatisfy myfelf on that point; when
I found the fineft *blob* of honey in her bladder,
exactly of the fame tafte, colour and fmell,
with that honey which is ufually collected
from fuch flowers as the bee was working u-
pon; for thofe bees which I picked off the
white clover, contained fine white tranfpar-
rent honey, while fuch as were taken from
heath, produced it of a high colour; and as
the honey had not been above a minute in
their bladders, it certainly could not undergo
any change in fo fhort a fpace of time. But
even allowing the bees their own ufual time to
collect, carry home, and depofit the honey in
their cells, the time will be found not to exceed five minutes; and yet the honey is, at
this period, in as great perfection, nay, rather
better, if there is any difference, than at any
time thereafter: for it is proved by experience,
and acknowledged by all connioffeurs in apiaries, that the younger the honey and honey-comb
are, they are fo much the fairer and better;
as, when they remain for fome time in the
hive, the combs, by the breath of the bees, gradually become of a darker colour, and the
honey becomes neither fo fair nor fo tranfpar-
rent,

rent, as when it was firſt collected*. From all
which conſiderations, it appears plain to me,
that bees are not the makers of honey, but only collectors of it ; and that the honey is in as
great perfection in the flowers, before the bees
touch it, if not better, than it is after it has paſ-
ſed through their bodies. †

* The author would not be underſtood here, as if he meant
that honey ſuddenly underwent a change to the worſe, as it will
remain many months locked up in the hives without undergoing
any material change ; yet, nevertheleſs, it is certain, that honey
is never better, than when it is newly depoſited in the cells.

† Some alledge, that the ſyrup in the flower, by paſſing
though the body of the bee, undergoes a material change, and
is thereby converted into real honey. But there is no analogy
between the honey extracted by the bee, to be carried home to
the hive, and the meant or drink taken into the ſtomach by any
other animal, to be digeſted for its nouriſhment. The former is
retained in the bladder of the bee only a few minutes ; whereas, the latter continues many hours, and, by the operation of
the gaſtric fluid, is changed into chyle, blood, &c. The honey
itſelf, when taken afterwards by the bees for the purpoſe of
nouriſhment, undergoes a ſimilar change ; but, in its firſt ſtate,
when put into the cells, it has undergone no change whatever.

I was this day favoured with a letter from a very intelligent
gentlemen, whoſe opinion, on this ſubject, although quite different from my own,—I ſhall preſent to my reader.

" Honey does not exiſt in the plant in that form, but only be-
" comes ſo by paſſing through the body of the bee. While it
" is in the flower, it conſtitutes what is called its ſaccharine
" juice

From the above reasoning we may conclude, that every single *heather bell*,* or cup of any other flower, is a vessel containing some of the finest honey, and that nothing in nature is a-wanting to make our land flow with it, and thereby enable both rich and poor to feast up-on it always at their pleasure.

A conjecture may naturally arise here, that, seeing bees do not *make* honey, but only col-lect it, if we could, by any device, fall upon a plan to extract it from the flowers; or, in o-ther words, to pour 10,000 of Nature's vessels full of honey into one of our artificial ones, it would be astonishing what a prodigious quan-tity might be produced throughout the island.

Scotland

" juice, and, when sucked up by the insect, is changed by the
" action of its vessels into honey.

": In proof of this assertion, take a number of hungry bees, and
" give them a full *meal* of sugar, diluted in water, tear one of
" them asunder immediately after, and its bladder will be found
" full of honey ; now, if sugar is so quickly converted into that
" form, have we any reason to doubt that the juice of the flower
" will undergo a change equally quick by the same means ?

" I have often made this experiment, and the result has been
" uniformly the same. If the bee has made a meal of white su-
" gar, the honey found in its body is white ; if it has got brown
" sugar or triacle, the honey will be brown."

* Flower of heath.

Scotland alone, I will venture to affirm, would,
in such a cafe, produce more honey and wax,
in one good feason, than would load one of his
Majesty's first rate men of war.   But as, hitherto, no fuch method has been difcovered, and
perhaps any fuch attempt would prove fruitlefs, let us ftudy to increafe, as quickly as poffible, the number of thofe *natural chemifts*, our
valuable, faithful, and induftrious fervants, the
BEES, who are every way qualified for the important tafk : having an exquifite fmell to direct them to the flowers containing the necta-
rine juice,—a *probofcis*, or fucking tube, to ena-
blé them to extract it,—a refervoir to contain
it,—wings to carry it away,—and fine clean
veffels of their own manufacture to treafure it
up in.   And let us ever deprecate the barbarous practice of deftroying fuch valuable creatures, who feem defigned by Nature to work
indefatigably for the benefit of mankind* ; and
therefore

---

* We cannot more ftrongly exprefs our deteftation of the
barbarous, and too general practice of fmoaking hives, than
in the beautiful and energetic language of the immortal
Thomfon :

Ah, fee where robb'd, and murder'd, in that pit
Lies the ftill heaving hive ! at evening fnatch'd,
Beneath the cloud of guilt concealing night,
And

therefore, inftead of death and extirpation, merit every encouragement and prefervation; and
ought, at leaft in autumn, to be allowed to re-
tain a reafonable fhare of the fruits of their
own induftry, to preferve them through the
D   winter

And fix'd o'er fulphur: while, not dreaming ill,
The happy people in their waxen cells,
Sat tending public cares, and planning fchemes
Of temperance, for Winter poor; rejoiced
To mark, full flowing round, their copious ftores.
Sudden the dark oppreffive fteam afcends;
And, uf'd to milder fcents, the tender race,
By thoufands, tumble from their honeyed domes,
Convolv'd, and agonizing in the duft.
And was it then for this you roam'd the Spring,
Intent from flower to flower? for this you toil'd
Ceafelefs the burning Summer-heats away?
For this in Autumn fearch'd the blooming wafte,
Nor loft one funny gleam? for this fad fate?
O Man! tyrannic lord! how long, how long,
Shall proftrate Nature groan beneath your rage,
Awaiting renovation? When obliged,
Muft you deftroy? Of their ambrofial food
Can you not borrow? and, in juft return,
Afford them fhelter from the wintry winds;
Or, as the fharp year pinches, with their own
Again regale them on fome fmiling day?
See where the ftony bottom of their town
Looks defolate, and wild; with here and there
A helplefs number, who the ruin'd ftate
Survive, lamenting, weak, caft out to death.

winter and fpring; whereby they will be enabled greatly to increafe in numbers, as well as
in produce, in the courfe of the fucceeding feafon.

In the next chapter we fhall take a view of
the vaft increafe of the number of hives that
may eafily be made in Scotland; an object
which I am happy to find already begins to
occupy the attention of many gentlemen of
property; and the promotion of which I hope
will foon become general. Nothing indeed
would yield me greater pleafure and fatisfaction, than if, by any exertion of mine, I could
be inftrumental in fetting on foot, or carrying
into execution, a meafure of fo much utility
and importance to the public.

C H A P. IV.

REASONS WHY THERE ARE SO FEW BEE-HIVES IN SCOTLAND.

IT is not to be expected, upon my propofed
plan, that I fhould enter deeply into the nature, generation, and properties of bees; although

though each of these subjects might afford an investigation equally useful and interesting. On such subjects, I have often thought, I could write a thousand pages, and, after all, be far from exhausting my thoughts on them. But, without diving deep at present into them, or entering the lists of controversy with other authors, who have wrote upon them, my chief design in this treatise was—

To excite men of property, who are the only proper persons to be addressed on the business, to exert themselves with spirit and perseverance to promote the increase of bee-hives in this country, by convincing them, that the cultivation of bees is an important object to the nation at large as well as to every proprietor of them.

To show, that the prices of HONEY and WAX would be thereby greatly reduced, and consequently these articles would become a source of national wealth ; and

That Britain, instead of expending large sums of money in purchasing these articles from foreign countries, might even be enabled to render them an article of exportation ; and therefore that they merit the attention of every patriot and real friend to his country. Also,

To

To show those who incline to make the attempt, how to proceed in such a laudable undertaking.

To give a brief account of the bee, as divided into its different classes of Queen, Drones, and Working bees; and to conclude with

Some plain and easy directions, how to manage that useful and industrious race, through the different seasons of the year, so as they may prove of the greatest advantage to the country at large, as well as to their proprietors.

The principal reason, why bees have not been reared in greater numbers in this country, is, the almost total neglect of them, by gentlemen of property; who seem, in general, to act as if they thought these useful insects entirely below their notice; and the rearing and increasing of bee-hives, as a business so very insignificant, as to be unworthy of their patronage. Hence many gentlemen will rather purchase honey at the highest rate, than give themselves the trouble of rearing bees; which neglect often likewise proceeds from an erroneous idea entertained by many, that bees will not thrive with them, and therefore the attempt would be fruitless. *

It

* Perhaps, in former ages, bees may have been more plentiful in Scotland,

It is not the want of proper pasture, that pre-vents bees from thriving well every year in this country. The only preventative is the in-constancy of the weather; for if it be windy, or cloudy, they will not go out of the hive; and, on the other hand, though the day should be quite dry, yet if the weather be cold, the bees will collect very little honey.

From all the above mentioned causes, therefore, it is plain, that the bees and the bee-master, have nothing so adverse to their interest as the mutability of the weather; and the worst of the matter is, that nothing can be done to re-medy this evil. Only the proprietor, by ha-ving plenty of good pasture at all seasons, has this advantage, that whatever good weather occurs between February and September, he may have his bees so well supplied with good flowers,

Scotland, than they have been for a considerable time past. This appears probable from different places still bearing their names from these useful animals. For instance, in my own native parish of Coldingham, there is a steeding called *Bee-Edge*, another named *Bee-Park*, and a rivulet denominated *Bee-Burn.* All these places have evidently derived their names from large quantities of bees having been formerly reared in them; as they are situat-ed on the skirts of a large common, which is now divided, and where bees would still thrive well with proper care and attention, if the proprietors would exert themselves to render these places worthy the names they bear.

flowers, as that they fhall be enabled to make
the moft of it, and to collect honey (as his hay-
makers make hay,) while the fun fhines. Here
it may be obferved, that bees will thrive well,
and collect a good quantity of honey in a fhort
time, if they only have three favourable days
in the week, during the honey feafon; as a
good hive, in thirty fine days, will collect four
pints of honey : befides, many people will alledge, that their fituation is too cold, windy,
or rainy, with many other reafons, which in
fact are of no weight; for the principal reafon
of bees not thriving is bad weather; and the
next chief caufe is the neglecting to take proper care of them. Their bees indeed will fometimes thrive long and well, with very little care,
which leads their proprietor to entertain an erroneous idea, that they always will do fo, and
that hardly any care is neceffary. But when
cold, famine, or robbing bees attack his hives,
and deftroy his ftock of bees, the lazy proprietor regrets his miftake when it is too late.

I believe poor people, in general, make more
by their bees annually, than thofe in more af-
fluent circumftances; and even the latter might
make far more of them than they do, if they
would only ftudy to increafe their ftock to a
confiderable

confiderable extent. The reafon is, that they are a kind of *eftate* to the poor, who, when once they enter upon the bufinefs of rearing bees, take a great pleafure in it, and, by paying proper attention to them, gradually acquire more and more knowledge in the profeffion. And, the only reafon why fuch perfons do not increafe their ftock of hives, to a much greater number than the country at prefent poffeffes, is, that pinching poverty obliges them often to fell the beft of their hives for ready money, to make up their houfe rent: Not to add, that fuch perfons, when obliged to leave their cottages, owing to raifed rents, monopolies of farms, or the like, think bee-hives a very troublefome fpecies of property for removal. Befides, as they keep but a few hives each, they never think of raifing any flowers for provifion to them. And if a perfon in fuch circumftances fhould lay out 20 s. for a hive, and fhe prove a bad one and die, he and fome of his neighbours will perhaps ever after look upon the culture of bees as a dangerous and precarious adventure, not to be attempted by any but perfons in affluence. To obviate fuch objections, fhall be the fubject of the following chapter.

CHAP.

CHAP. V.

REASONS FOR, AND PRACTICABILITY OF, INCREASING THE NUMBER OF BEE-HIVES IN SCOTLAND.

A NY perfon, who confiders how very abundantly Scotland is fupplied by nature, with food proper for bees, throughout almoft every county in the kingdom, and obferves how very few bees are reared, notwithftanding thefe great advantages, muft be furprifed that fo little exertion has hitherto been made in that line. For inftance, were we to confider, that fome parifhes, which might abundantly maintain 300 hives in each of them, have not at prefent 20 or 30, we muft be furprized at that infatuation which has hitherto prevented us from attending more to our own intereft. Were we to confider our large extended heath-covered moors, and beautiful clover fields, with the great quantities of runches, wild muftard, &c. that grow fpontaneoufly in our corn fields,

together

gether with the many elegant gardens, nurferies, &c. raifed by art, in the neighbourhood
of this metropolis, and almoft every other town
in Scotland, as well as the country feats of our
gentry, together with thofe numerous wild flowers that grow in our meadow grounds and
pafture lands, we might juftly fay, " the HAR-
" VEST truly is GREAT, but the LABOURERS
" are FEW."

And here I fhall mention a thought, which
ftruck me lately in a gentleman's garden, and
indeed has often ftruck me in fimilar fituations ;—" Here I am furrounded with a variety of fine flowers, and the profpect all a-
round me is equally pleafant and delightful!
What a variety of Nature's beauties and fweets
are here exhibited, and how many thoufands
of millions of fockets of flowers there are, in
the vaft number of gardens in this metropolis
and its environs !—and yet, the infatuated inhabitants and proprietors rather allow the
honey contained in thefe beautiful veffels to
be wafted, than employ a few of thofe faithful fervants, provided by nature, to extract
and collect it for them :—Servants, who would
chearfully labour, without wages, and find
themfelves in food and cloathing during their

E   employment

employment, if the proprietor would only provide them a few fmall lodgings. Will thefe people ftill rather be at the expence of purchafing honey from me, or others, at a high rate, than rear hives to manufacture it for themfelves? Will they continue to fend their money to Dantzick, for honey of a far inferior quality, rather than encourage the produce of it at home?—Why do not the gentry of Edinburgh and the neighbourhood, efpecially thofe who live in the confines of the city, replenifh their gardens and nurferies with fome hundreds of hives, which they are fo well able to fill?" Similar reflections have often ftruck my mind, when I have feen extenfive fields, abounding with white clover and heath, where the flowers, like the ftars of heaven, or the fand on the fea fhore, could be numbered not by units, tens, hundreds, or thoufands, but by *millions*!—Suppofe, for example, 1 fquare yard of heath or clover to contain 500 cups of flowers, each one of which contains fome honey, what an immenfe number would be contained in an extent of 6 fquare miles?

Some however here may reply, that a field may be overftocked with bees, as well as with fheep or black cattle. I will grant that there

is

is a poffibility of this, but I will venture to affirm, that fuch a thing has feldom ever yet happened in Britain*. Or, at leaft, if there is, or
ever was, any one place in the ifland overftocked with them, there are twenty other places, which never reared the fourth part of
the number that they were able to maintain.
Nay, there are many excellent fituations for
bees, which perhaps never had 20 ftock hives
on them, although by nature abundantly provided with excellent pafture for many hun-
E 2 *   dreds.

* There are fome few places, indeed, fuch as white benty
ground, where there is fcarcely a heath, clover, muftard, or
runch flower to be feen, nor even any furze, broom, or plane
trees growing, and which are almoft quite void of all other flowers. Such places are certainly very bad fituations for bees, and
they will never thrive on them, or on any fimilar unproductive
grounds. There are again fome other places, which have but a
few natural flowers, and where no artificial ones are reared. Such
places may perhaps have hardly a fufficient quantity of flowers in
eight miles circumference, to feed eight ftocks of hives ; Whereas, in more favourable fituations, the fame extent of ground
could eafily produce as many flowers as would feed eight fcore.
There are fome other grounds, which are excellent for producing corn, but which perhaps have little clover, muftard, or runches, in their neighbourhood, and neither gardens nor moors within reach. Such places are naturally bad fituations for bees ; but
by rearing fome turnips, muftard, or clover, and fome furze in
hedges, or on wafte grounds, they may eafily be rendered excellent fituations for thefe ufeful infects.

dreds.   For, as has been often mentioned, when
we confider the vaft quantity of flowers, which
the earth naturally produces, and which might
be ftill much more increafed by art, how pro-
digiously great may we eftimate the total?
This confideration may convince us of the little
danger we have of running into the extreme
of overftocking our fields with bees.

Some may perhaps alledge, that if there were
twenty times more hives in Scotland than there
are at prefent, the produce, in a bad feafon,
would ftill be very trifling : But this is a very
childifh objection ; for, even in the worft of feafons, the quantity of honey produced, would,
by proper care and attention, ftill be twenty
times greater than, in fuch a feafon, it is at
prefent.   For inftance, were there but one hive
in all Scotland, in a cold rainy fummer ; even
that hive would produce but a very fmall increafe, perhaps fwarm only once, and that fwarm
produce but only one pint of honey ; whereas,
if there are 100 hives, granting the weather to
be equally bad, the produce muft be at leaft
100 pints of honey.   Eftimating the number
of parifhes in Scotland, capable of raifing bees,
to be only 800, which I think is below the
truth, the following calculation will give a view

of

of the immenſe quantity of honey that might be produced, even in ordinary favourable years.

	Hives.		*Pints of Honey.*
Suppoſing, (which is moderate)	1	to produce	4
Then 1 hive in each pariſh -	800	produces	3,200
Suppoſing the number in each pariſh increaſed to 30, -	24,000	will produce	96,000
But ſuppoſing, (which is ſtill very moderate) the number in each pariſh increaſed to 100 · - - -	80,000	will produce	320,000
Suppoſing the number in each pariſh increaſed to 400 -	320,000	will produce	1,280,000

			lbs. of wax.
Beſides wax, which at 1lb. each hive, is	-	-	80,000

But there are many pariſhes in Scotland ſo very large and extenſive, and ſo full of rich flowers, that I believe 1000 hives erected in each of them, would not contain bees ſufficient to extract the one half of the honey contained in their flowers, in favourable weather; and therefore, it would not be eſtimating the poſſible increaſe of honey, all over Scotland, too high, to ſtate it at near 2,000,000 of pints of honey. For example, the pariſh in which I reſide, was ſo richly provided laſt year with abundance of fine white clover, wild muſtard, and heath flowers, &c. that 1500 hives of bees, placed properly on it, would not have nearly

exhauſted

exhaufted its flowers of their honey. To what an aftonifhing extent then might the bee-huf-bandry be carried ? *

But left I fhould be thought extravagant, in my calculations and ftatements of the profits to be made from thefe ufeful animals, and in-clined to lead my readers to build *caftles in the air*, inftead of erecting hives in their gardens, I fhall mention a few facts out of many on this fubject, which I can vouch, either from my own concern in them, or upon the autho-rity of perfons with whom I am particularly acquainted, and who informed me how much they had made of their bees laft feafon.

To a perfon near Greenlaw, I
   paid for honey and wax, a-
   bove,   -   -   -   L. 4   0   0
To another near Dunfe, for
   ditto, above,   -   -   11   0   0
To another, near Hamilton, I
   paid for *one hive*, which was
   weighed in the Edinburgh
   Weigh-houfe,   -   -   4   0   0

For

* But it is neceffary to caution the reader here, that, in a very bad feafon, it perhaps could do little more than produce the fourth part of that quantity; not for want of abundance of flow-ers with honey in them, but for want of favourable weather for them to go and collect it. See pages 7, 9 and 29.

For 40 hives, purchafed from
    different perfons, fome of
    them at above 2l. Sterling
    each, I paid   -   -   70 0 0
A friend in Mid-Lothian af-
    fured me, he had cleared laft
    feafon, by his bees, no lefs
    than   -   -   -   12 0 0

All of thefe perfons had but a very few
ftock hives at Whitfunday, and yet they made,
at an average, above 30s. by each of their hives.
But had they increafed their ftock, they might
eafily have made ten times more than they
did.

With regard to the profit arifing from bees,
one confideration fhould not be overlooked,
viz. that almoft the whole produce, arifing from
the fale of both honey and wax, is in a great
meafure clear profit; as bees, and bee-hives
are, particularly in Scotland, equally free from
rents and taxes; and the culture of them does
not in the leaft injure or impede any other improvement, in any refpeᴄt. Nor do they require a conftant attendance, as moft other articles of improvement do; for a proper perfon
might eafily overfee, with a little affiftance in
fwarming time, at leaft 500 bee-hives. And.

aᴢ

as Nature has amply fupplied them with food, and with powers to provide it for themfelves, they put their owners to little or no expence for that article; which cannot be faid of any other of our fervants whatever.*

Thus, by following the above plan, with a little attention and exertion on the part of our landed gentlemen, fuch a number of bee-hives would foon be raifed all over the kingdom, that

* Here I have in view Scotland in general, as it has many hundreds of fituations where bees would thrive well, but where not a fingle flower is fown for that purpofe; but even were this plan adopted, of rearing artificial flowers in thofe places, where a fcarcity of natural flowers prevails, during part of the working feafon, in order to fupply that defect, and thus afford the bees abundance of provifion at all times, ftill the expence would be fo trifling, that it is fcarcely worth taking notice of; as is already hinted, p. 12, &c. for, fhould we plant fome trees, with a view to affift bees, we have their wood; if we rear turnips, we have their feed; if we fow white clover, we have the beft of pafture; and if we even allow furze or broom to overfpread wafte grounds, we can be at little lofs, as even thefe have alfo their ufes, by fupplying us with hedging, fuel, fhelter for fheep, &c. I wifh not to be here underftood, as if I meant to recommend the fowing of large fields purpofely with food for bees, excepting white clover, which provides food for larger animals: All that I intend is, that gentlemen, who have great ftocks of bees, and plenty of ground, may eafily fpare three or four acres, out of as many hundreds, for the rearing of turnips, muftard, furze, broom, &c.

that the quantity of honey and wax would be increased to such an extent, as to produce the greatest advantages to the nation at large, as well as to the private proprietors of the hives. All the money sent to foreign markets for these commodities would be kept at home; which would be a saving of perhaps not less than 50,000l. a-year. And honey would be produced in such abundance at home, as to supply the poor, as well as the rich, not only with a delicious *luxury*, but also with an excellent substitute for some *necessaries.*

It might, for instance, be converted into *mead*, a fine well-tasted wholesome liquor, which would prove an excellent substitute for strong ale and porter, and could be sold at a very moderate price. A weaker kind of mead, called *bragwort*, could also be made of it. This is an agreeable wholesome liquor, much esteemed by many, who use it as a substitute for small beer. When properly made, it will keep long: And when of a proper degree of strength, it is so highly exhilarating, that many persons have been sent home half intoxicated with it.

The increase of the quantity of honey would also reduce the price of it so much, that in-

F   stead

stead of paying 10d. or 1s. *per* pound for it, as at present, it might be sold so low as 3d. *per* pound, in which case it would prove an excellent substitute for butter to the poor. Even at the present prices, it is already used by many persons mixed with butter.

As to the wax, almost every person knows the great uses made of that article, in medicinal preparations, wax candles, sealing wax, &c. &c. as well as the high esteem in which wax candles and wax tapers, are held by persons in the higher ranks of life, on account of their clear light and odoriferous smell, as well as their freedom from all danger of greasing any thing, as tallow candles do, when a drop falls from them.

CHAP.

CHAP. VI.

HOW TO INCREASE THE NUMBER OF BEE-HIVES IN A FEW YEARS IN SCOTLAND.

I PROCEED next to show, in what manner the number of bee-hives may be speedily encreased in Scotland. If a gentleman of property has a proper situation for bees, and the above reasoning has inclined him to commence the cultivation of bees with spirit, let him apply to some person tolerably skilled in that branch of science, and let him purchase 100 or more bee-hives, in the month of August, and place them properly, according to the directions which shall be laid down hereafter. Let him next rear a sufficiency of turnips in their neighbourhood, that they may blossom next spring; and in the month of February, let him sow some mustard seed, and some furze and broom upon dykes, or waste ground. Gentlemen of property, who have any ground proper for planting, should by all means plant a number

F 2   of

of plane trees and fallows. They fhould likewife fow a good deal of white clover, fweet
refida, or mignionette, &c. with any other
flowers that will grow upon the ground, either
by nature or art.

In winter, particular care fhould be taken to
preferve the bees from cold; in fpring, from
~~famine,~~ and robbery by other bees. And
when they are ready to fwarm, great care muft
be taken to lodge them in proper habitations.

With fuch attentive management, I can venture to affure all who will make the experiment,
that 100 well-chofen ftock-hives, will, in a tolerably good feafon, produce from 180 to
200 or even 220 hives, whatever more.

Some may object, that, while the proprietor, who wifhes to increafe the breed of bees,
raifes many flowers for that purpofe, his
neighbour, who, perhaps, takes no trouble of
this kind, may fhare the benefit, by his bees
coming and feeding upon them §.   To this it
may

§ I was fent for on the 23d of May laft, by a gentleman in
Edinburgh, who wifhed me to bring him a hive of bees, and to
pitch upon the moft proper fituation for placing it in his garden.
The day being very fine, and the fruit trees in full bloffom,
there was a pear tree among many others, which was full of fine
bloffoms: Obferving a number of bees bufily employed upon
them,

be fufficient to reply, that the induſtrious proprietor, having done every thing in his power to
                                fupply

them, he told me, " they belonged to his *neighbour*, who lived
" a few yards from him."—" Perhaps not," replied I, " for a
" bee will fly far for food in fine weather : and, therefore, thefe
" bees may come from Leith, or fome other place as far diſtant,
" while your neighbour's bees may fly as far as Leith for their
" loading."

As for the reafon why bees will fometimes travel a mile or
more for a heavy loading, when they could get the fame quantity and equally good, from the fame fpecies of flowers within a
few yards, I can fcarcely hazard a conjecture ; unlefs it be, that
perhaps fome of the old and experienced bees, from a miſtaken
apprehenfion, may fuppofe thofe flowers near their hives to have
been exhauſted, by the moſt part of the hive having had conſtant
accefs to them, and feeding on them ; as is faid of the old cattle,
that they commonly feed on the borders of their pafture grounds,
where few of the younger cattle have previoufly fed. But, as a
proof of the fact, let any perfon who has one or two hives, with a-
bundance of flowers to keep his bees conſtantly employed, within
100 yards of their hives, make the experiment, by going to another place, where there are alfo flowers growing 1000 yards diftant from his own, or any other perfons bees, and he will find a
great number of bees at work on the diſtant flowers.

But though fome bees, by being expeditious travellers, feem to
difregard diſtance, and to be fond of undertaking long journeys
even when loaded, yet, in general, I believe, the greater part
of them are wife enough to collect their loading as near their
hives as poffible. And, therefore, the nearer the flowers are fituated, the more work will they perform, and the greater quantity of honey will be carried home in a day. For this reafon, I
have already advifed the hives to be always placed as near as
poffible to plenty of provifions.

supply his own bees with ample provisions, will
have the pleasure to see them feed and thrive
upon it; and should those of his neighbours
occasionally partake, he will not have any reason to regard it, there being no danger of a
famine. But to obviate this objection completely, let ten (or more) persons in a village,
or neighbourhood, join together and contribute
equally in proportion to the number of their
hives, to rear a sufficient quantity of flowers a-
mongst them, and upon this amicable plan, the
expence of each proprietor will be exactly in
proportion to the number of his hives.

Supposing, that there are, in May 1795,
twenty stock hives in each parish in Scotland,
the amount in 800 parishes would be 16,000.
Then, supposing each of these hives to throw
one swarm, which would probably keep through
the winter, in September we would have 32000
stock hives. At this period, let every gentleman, who rears bees, keep all his hives, young
and old, for stock hives, that are fit for it*:
Let

---

* All stocks, or first swarms, and even some second swarms, will
probably answer for that purpose; and all swarms which are nearly full of combs, but rather light, such as I would not advise to be
kept, if they were not speedily to increase the stock; by keeping
them

Let the poor, who are able, do the fame with theirs ;—and let thofe, who are not able to lie out of the produce of their bees, fell them to thofe who are inclined to purchafe them for ftock hives. By doing this, they will raife as much honey as if they killed all the bees, and fold the honey and wax†, and with far lefs trouble.

On thefe principles, by keeping 32,000 ftock hives, with proper management, during a tolerable feafon, and always preferving all that will preferve, for the fpace of feven years, the ftock would increafe as follows : viz.

HIVES.

them, and feeding carefully with courfe honey, which might be purchafed from any foreign market, where it could be got at the cheapeft rate. For this purpofe, two or three very light fwarms, which are not fit to be kept for ftocks feparately, might, by conjoining both bees and honey, form a good ftock hive. And all hives, containing honey or combs, whofe bees defert them from whatever caufe, during any feafon of the year, might be kept carefully, to lodge new fwarms next feafon. The method of uniting, feeding, &c. will be defcribed in their proper places ; and by following the directions laid down under thefe heads, our hives would in a fhort time turn out very numerous.

† But fhould it here be afked, How are we to be fupplied with honey during the time of rearing the ftock hives ? we may reply, that it may be purchafed from other counties, in order to fupply ourfelves, as well as to feed our weak hives.

	HIVES.
In the 1. year, Sept. 1795, there would be	32,000
———— 2. ——— —— 1796, ————————	64,000
———— 3. ——— —— 1797, ————————	128,000
———— 4. ——— ——— 1798, ————————	256,000
———— 5. ——— ——— 1799, ————————	512,000
———— 6. ——— ——— 1800, ————————	1,024,000
———— 7. ——— ——— 1801, ————————	2,048,000

Thus, within the fhort period of feven years, the number of our bee-hives would be increafed to no lefs than TWO MILLIONS and FORTY EIGHT THOUSAND HIVES. But allowing the forty eight thoufand to be difcounted for dead hives, there would ftill remain two millions of ftock hives. Although this number may appear to be large, yet there is no reafon to fuppofe, that the calculation is neither impoffible or improbable. But, even dropping the one half of this number, upon the fuppofition of loffes by bad feafons, &c. there would ftill remain, at the loweft eftimate, a clear MILLION of ftock hives; which, next year might produce FOUR MILLIONS of PINTS of HONEY, and ONE MILLION of POUNDS of WAX; and ftill keeps the ftock entire. With fuch a quantity, indeed, of thefe ufeful animals, and valuable commodities, we might reft contented; as fuch a quantity, befides every other advantage, would afford employment to hundreds of old

and

and poor people to watch them in fwarming time, and to make hives to receive the young colonies.

Another method, by which the number of our ftock hives may be more fpeedily increafed in this country, might eafily be adopted. Should any one opulent proprietor, or a company of individuals, incline to have 2000 or 3000 bee-hives, let a commiffion be fent by a proper perfon to Poland or Ruffia, where, in the month of Auguft efpecially, they could be purchafed at one third part of the price they generally draw here: And I am perfuaded, if the Dantzick hives are made much in the fame form with ours, or in any other form that will admit of carriage, a fhip nearly loaded with other goods, which would help to pay her freight, might bring over a great number of them. Perhaps many will think this an extravagant attempt, but I am fo confident of its fuccefs, that if I were poffeffed of 1000 l. Sterling in ready cafh, I would fet fail for Dantzick, and rifk 800 l. of it upon the adventure. On bringing home my cargo of living bees, I would fpread them all over the kingdom: But, before fetting out upon fuch a voyage, I would firft inform myfelf properly about

G the

the form of the Dantzick hives, as well as about their prices, and whether they are to be got near the fea-coaft; as land carriage of bees is equally trdublefome, expenfive, and dange- rous: But I would not be afraid to rifk 1000 bee-hives on board a fhip; for, I would rather carry them 4000 miles on fhip-board, when properly packed, than 100 by land.

C H A P. VII.

ACCOUNT OF THE QUEEN BEE.

THE QUEEN, or MOTHER BEE, is eafily diftinguifhed from all the other bees in the hive, by the form, fize, and colour of her body. She is confiderably longer, and her wings are much fhorter in proportion to her body, than thofe of the other bees. The wings of both common bees and drones, cover their whole bodies, whereas thofe of the Queen fcarce reach beyond the middle, ending about the third ring of her belly. Her hinder part is

far

far more tapering than those of the other bees: Her belly and legs are yellower, and her upper parts of a much darker colour, than theirs. She is also furnished with a sting, though some authors assert that she has none, having been induced to form this opinion, because she is extremely pacific; so much so, indeed, that one may handle her, and even teaze her as much as he pleases, without provoking her resentment. For my part, I never could excite a Queen Bee to draw her sting, nor could I even get a sight of it, but when I pressed her body. The omniscient Governor of Nature has wisely ordained this majestic insect to be of a pacific disposition; for, were she otherwise,—were she, like the other bees, of so irritable a temper as to draw her sting on every occasion, and to leave it in the body of her antagonist, it would prove of dangerous and often fatal consequences to the whole hive; for every bee, after losing her sting, dies within a day or two at the utmost.

· The Queen bee is solemn and calm in her deportment. A young Queen is a great deal smaller in size than a full grown one; being not much longer than a common bee, and is therefore not so easily observed when sought for.

G 2   When

When only three or four days old, she is very quick in her motions, and runs very fast; but when pregnant with eggs, she becomes very large, and her body is heavy. When travelling, she drags along in a very flow manner, and is not very expeditious in flying. It is proper that every proprietor of bees should know the Queen, as it may often be of great advantage to him. The surest way to know her is to get a sight of one from some acquaintance, who keeps hives: or, if this cannot be obtained, he may search for her, by the above description, among some small hives.

That this majestic animal is a female, the very designation she bears, of QUEEN, seems to imply that all modern authors are convinced, though many of the ancients were of a different opinion. But as it is also now unanimously admitted, that she lays every egg in the hive, she ought rather to be called the MOTHER BEE. For, indeed, from the best observation that ever I could make, she possesses and exerts NO SOVEREIGNTY over the other bees. She evidences the greatest anxiety for the good of the commonwealth, with which she is connected; and, indeed, every member of it shows an equal regard for her welfare. But I never could observe,

ferve, that fhe iffues any pofitive orders, to be
punctually obeyed by the other bees. The
truth feems to be, that fhe and the other bees
are all equally acquainted with their duty by
iuftinct, and have an equal pleafure in performing it, without waiting for orders from each
other. That there is, neverthelefs, the greateft
order and regularity among them, is certain;
for they lay their plans and execute them in
the beft poffible manner, by the influence of
the above powerful fubftitute for reafon.

Almoft all writers, as formerly hinted, are
of opinion, that the Queen lays three different
kinds of eggs; viz. one kind for the production of a Queen Bee; another fpecies for that
of the working bees, and a third for producing
the Drones. It was alfo long a received opinion,
that no Queen could lay eggs, that were capable of producing bees, without the affiftance of
Drones. SCHIRACH †, on this fubject, refutes
this doctrine, and entirely denies fuch an ufe
of the Drones. He advances this opinion, that
" the Queen lays eggs, which produce young
" bees, without any communication with the
Drones;

† Paftor of KLEIN BAUTZEN, in UPPER LUSATIA, and Secretary
to a Society of Naturalifts there.

" Drones; and affirms that all the working
" bees are females in difguife; every one of
" whom, in an early ftage of her exiftence, was
" capable of becoming a Queen; from a know-
" ledge of which fact, fwarms may artificially
" be obtained from the early months of fpring,
" and in any fucceeding month, even to No-
" vember."

His experiments have been very numerous,
and obviate every doubt and objection. He
performed the operation, upon one and the
fame ftock, for at leaft fifty or fixty times, from
mere fragments of the combs, &c. &c. This
novel and wonderful doctrine excited no fmall
contention, and not a few counter experiments
among naturalifts on the Continent, without
being decided even by the great BONNET. He
afferts, which is indeed the grand and decifive
proof, that " the practice of this art, (of rai-
" fing artificial Queens,) has already extended
" itfelf through Upper Lufatia, the Palatinate,
" Bohemia, Bavaria, Silefia, and feveral parts of
" Germany, and even of Poland."

That a Queen can be raifed from an egg in
a common cell, or, in other words, that the
felf-fame egg is capable of being reared up to
be either a Queen, or a common bee, as the

bees

bees pleafe, appears to´me, from my own experiments, to be paft a doubt; and that a Queen, who never faw a drone, can lay eggs, which will produce bees, is equally certain. Both of thefe facts will, I flatter myfelf, appear to the curious and learned reader, to be clearly afcertained by the following experiments.

Long before I heard of Mr Schirach's theory, or experiments, I had often taken off fwarms, without leaving any Queens or royal cells in the mother hive; notwithftanding which, they bred young Queens, which furprized me greatly how they had obtained them, as the received opinion then was, that they could not breed a Queen bee, if the old Queen was taken away, before a royal cell was erected. But after feeing Schirach's fentiments on this fubject, I thought his theory extremely probable, according to what I had obferved among my own bees; and refolving to afcertain the truth of it, I made many experiments of my own, which all fucceeded to my wifhes. But, in order to put the matter beyond all doubt, I fhall relate an experiment I made with a hive in fpring 1788, two months before the ufual time of fwarming, and which clearly afcertains both the facts at once. The hive

was

was beginning to carry well, and to breed faft, but it was not half full of bees. It had only one Queen, but neither Drone nor royal cell ; neither of which could be expected at that feafon of the year, as it was about the middle of April. I took out the Queen, and moft part of the bees, and left the hive with only fome common bees, to hatch out the young brood in the cells, and provide themfelves with a Queen, but without leaving one fingle Drone. They did not difappoint me; for as foon as the melancholy intelligence pervaded the hive, that their loving mother was torn from them, they made a mourning kind of noife for their great lofs, for about two hours : After which, a general council, as it would feem, being called, the moft experienced fages, in the diftreffed republic, may be fuppofed to have advifed their brethren, " That it was in vain to mourn longer for the lofs of their mother and brothers; that although they were gone, and although they had at prefent no royal cell to raife another mother, yet they had ftill fufficient refources from nature and their own induftry; that they had power and means to raife a young monarch to the throne; that they had plenty of new laid eggs, and there-

fore

fore no time was to be loft, to raife a Queen
bee from one of them; otherwife the eggs
would all foon produce common bees, and
then all hopes of future progeny would ceafe
for ever, and their republic utterly perifh, for
want of a prolific mother to preferve and per-
petuate the race."

That the bees feemed to have had fome
fuch reafoning among them, appeared pretty
evident from their conduct; for about two
hours after the capture of the Queen, they all
fell bufily to work, and exerted themfelves a-
mazingly for two days; fome being employed in forming the royal cell, and others in in-
jecting into it a large quantity of thick whitifh liquid ftuff, pretty much refembling cream.
At the end of the 3d day, the royal cell was
completely formed; and, in the mean time,
the common cells were fealed up by the other
bees, who all continued bufily employed.
On the fifth day, the royal cell was confiderably enlarged, and I obferved as much of the a-
forefaid white ftuff in it, as would have half filled a thimble almoft, with a white maggot lying
on the top of it On the feventh day, the bees
fealed it up, and, on the feventeenth day, the
young Queen came forth out of her little pa-

H   lace

lace, in all her pomp and majefty. On the twenty-fourth day, the young Queen became a MOTHER, and laid eggs; on the thirty-firft day, thefe eggs were fealed up, and, on the forty-third day, a number of young bees emerged from the cells. About the fame time I repeated this experiment with other two hives, which both fucceeded equally well.

I made another experiment with a different hive, out of which I took the Queen and moft part of the bees. This hive had neither a royal cell nor drones in it, yet, in feventeen days thereafter, a Queen was reared, and on the 25th day fhe laid eggs. I then took out the young Queen again, leaving fome new laid eggs in the old hive. Within eight days after, there was another royal cell erected and fealed up. This I immediately took out of the hive; but, upon infpecting the hive eight days thereafter, I found neither Queen, eggs, nor royal cell, none of which indeed I expected. Upon taking a piece of comb, however, with eggs in it, out of another hive, and putting it into this hive, the bees erected another royal cell, which in due time produced another young Queen.

The advocates for the doctrine of the drones being males, and their aid being neceffary for the

the propagation of bees, may perhaps plead,
that although there were no drones in the hive,
when I took the Queen from it, yet there
might have been eggs laid in drone cells, which
would come forward to be drones as foon as
the young Queen, and fo impregnate her, and
render her fit for breeding. But the contrary
is the fact : for, when the old Queen was taken
out of the hive, there was not a fingle egg in
any of the drone cells. If there had, I would
have feen the bees fitting upon the cells of the
drone combs, as they did on thofe of the
common bees, and on the royal cell. Befides,
I turned up the hive every fecond day, during
the whole period of forty-three days, in order
to determine how long the bees took to erect
the royal cell, and feal it up ; how many days
elapfed before an egg produced a Queen ; how
old the Queen was, before fhe began to lay
eggs ; how many days pafled, before thefe eggs
produced common bees ; and, above all, whether the Queen needed the agency of the
drones, to enable her to become a mother.
To arrive at a certainty on this point, I often
turned the bees over in the hive with a fmall
ftick, in fearch of young drones in drone
cells, but could not difcover the fmalleft vef-

H 2 tige

tige of them. But the young Queen, on the
10th day of her age, began to lay eggs in
drone cells, which produced young Drones in
the hive about sixteen days thereafter. Having repeated this last experiment again and a-
gain, I can now affirm, with the utmost confidence and certainty, that the common, or
working bees, are endowed with the powerful
faculty of raising a Queen bee, from an egg,
in a common cell, when their community
stands in need of one.

Their method is this: They make choice
of a common cell with an egg in it, and inject some white liquid matter, from their proboscis, of a thickish substance. They then
begin to build upon the edges of the cell, and
enlarge it. On the third day, it appears fairly
on the outside of the comb, in the form of a
royal cell, and may now be properly so denominated. On the fifth day, the cell being now
greatly enlarged, and a great deal of the whitish matter thrown into it, the royal maggot
appears in the form of a semicircle, not unlike
a new moon, being biggest in the middle part,
and small at each end. In this form it is to
be seen for two days, swimming on the top,

and

and in the midſt of the ſaid matter in the cell ; and on the ſeventh day it is ſealed up.

During this period, our young princeſs undergoes various metamorphoſes. I have opened the royal cell on the tenth day, and have found the maggot ſtill on the top of the white liquor ; and having taken it into my hand to ſhow it to any friend, it would have moved for a ſhort time, although at this period, it had not the ſmalleſt reſemblance to a bee, being ſtill only a maggot. But on the fourteenth or fifteenth day, the metamorphoſis is ſo complete, that inſtead of a groſs white worm, forth comes a charming young Queen Bee, † arrayed in all her glory. From the whole of theſe experiments, therefore, which I have repeated on various occaſions, I can poſitively affirm, that the Qeen Bee is capable of becoming a mother, without ſo much as ſeeing a drone ; and that the

---

† The ſame proceſs, or nearly ſo, is uſed by the common bees, to bring forward both their own ſpecies and drones, by throwing the whitiſh matter on the eggs, and ſealing them up, till the maggots undergo the uſual changes in the cells, &c. And each egg generally produces a bee in about fourteen or ſixteen days. I have ſeen them differ two or three days in point of time. Perhaps an egg, ſhould the bees let it alone and inject no matter upon it, might, nevertheleſs, keep warm for 8 days, and produce a bee at laſt,

the doctrines of almost all former writers on this
subject, (Schirach and one or two more except-
ed,) who affirm that the Queen cannot breed
without the agency of the drones, or males,
as they call them, is founded on a mistake.
For a small piece of comb, with common eggs
in it, may be taken and put into a box along
with 400 common bees, and transported 1000
miles from a Drone; and yet the bees will rear
a Queen from one of those eggs, and that young
Queen will lay eggs, which in due time will
produce Queens, commons and drones. But
whether every egg in the common cells of the
hive can be nourished up to produce a Queen,
I dare not positively say; although I am much
inclined to think so, as I can safely affirm, that
not above one in a dozen of my experiments, in
rearing Queens from what are called *common
eggs*, (i. e. eggs that commonly produce working
bees,) has ever yet failed, when I either made
the trial by way of experiment, or adopted the
plan as a matter of œconomy.   Sometimes a
single egg has failed in making the experiment;
but this might have happened from some other
accidental cause. As a proof of this, I offer to
rear 20 Queens, if not 30, out of one hive, during the course of one summer.   For I have,
                                    within

within thefe laft fix years, caufed the bees to
rear, from eggs taken from common cells, which
the bees would otherwife have reared up
for working bees, no fewer than 200 *artificial*
Queens; and which Queens laid eggs, that
came forward to be bees, in the fame manner
as other Queens, which may, for diftinction's
fake, be ftiled *natural* ones.

Sometimes, when I have taken the Queen out
of a hive, and left none but common bees in
it, after looking for the fpace of fourteen or
fixteen days, for royal cells, as ufual in fuch
cafes, I have obferved, that, inftead of Queens
being produced, there were three or four royal cells, which contained nothing in them, except that fome of them had a red tough matter, of a hard kind of fubftance, about the fize of
a pea, which would tear, but would not break:
while others of them would have contained neither egg, maggot, nor chryfalis, but were quite
empty. Thefe empty cells I fhall, for diftinction's fake, call *falfe royal cells.* What was the
intention of the bees, in rearing thefe falfe royal
cells, I cannot determine. The bees were furely fenfible, that there were no young bees in
them: and yet they would have allowed them
to

to continue in the hive for many months. One circumstance inclines me to think, that the bees intended them to be of some use for rearing Queens, as I never saw these false royal cells reared, but when the hive wanted a Queen. I am equally certain, however, on the other hand, that I have never once seen an egg or decayed maggot in any of them. I own that some common cells will sometimes be sealed up, as if there were young bees in them, although none would ever appear. All of these, however, had eggs in them at first, which had decayed and rotten, by cold or some other accident. But this I never found to be the case, in those false royal cells, not one of which appeared to have ever had one in them. Therefore, when we leave a hive without a Queen, we cannot positively say, that the bees will rear one for themselves : yet were the practice eligible in every other respect, we might trust to it, as scarcely one case in a dozen fails. But if a royal cell, on the 2d, 3d, or 4th day, after it is erected, appear to have an egg, or some of the whitish matter in it, a Queen may be depended upon, to be produced in due time, if no accident prevent.

That

That the Queen and the common or working bees are of the same sex in the egg, and yet
that they can rear up bees of every species between them, appears to me to be no more
wonderful than true *. Whether the additional matter thrown into the enlarged cell, along
with the egg, is of a generative or nutritive nature, I cannot yet positively determine, altho'
I rather incline to think it is of the former
kind.—But there are considerable difficulties
on both sides. For, if we say the white matter
is of a generative quality, then we must suppose that the working bees are males ; although
it must appear very unaccountable, that the
same egg should be capable of rearing either a
male or a *female*, at the option of the working
bees :—which, however, upon this supposition,

I   appears

* Whether the bees can rear up one of those eggs that are
laid in drone cells, to become a Queen or a common bee; or
whether they can rear eggs that have been laid in common cells,
to become drones, is not yet ascertained. This question, however, might easily be decided, by putting a piece of comb with
drone eggs in it, along with 400 common bees ; and, by repeating the experiment 6 or 8 times, it might soon be discovered,
whether the bees could raise one of those drone eggs to be a
Queen bee. I rather incline to think, that the eggs laid in
drone cells cannot be raised to be any other but drone bees,
and that those laid in common cells can never be reared to become drones.

appears clearly proved, by Schirach's experiments and my own. On the other hand, if we hold it to be of a nutritive nature, then we suppose the Queen to be a hermaphrodite, or *self-prolific*, without the assistance of any other creature. It is indeed reported, that the whole genus of snails are hermaphrodites, and that each individual of the species is endued with both sexes.

But although I have not a doubt as to the fact, that an egg in a common cell is capable of being nourished up to produce a Queen, yet I rather doubt, whether any great improvement can be made of this discovery, so as to increase the quantity of honey and wax; as it is not a great number of hives that will produce that effect, but only real good ones. I also doubt, whether more hives can be reared by this method, as our bees generally produce more Queens naturally, than they are able to supply with a sufficient number of common bees to compose a proper swarm with; as appears from their killing the supernumerary ones, which they have no need of.—Often, for instance, in a garden containing four stock hives in May, they will breed perhaps 24 Queens during the summer, but will kill two thirds of them, and send off
the

the other 8, with as many young fwarms.—It muft be allowed, however, that hives will fometimes ly long out; and, therefore, if the owner had a fpare Queen, he might eafily rear new fwarms with them, which he cannot fafely do without them.

C H A P. VIII.

ACCOUNT OF THE DRONE BEE.

THE DRONES are a fpecies of bees, well known to every Bee-mafter, and may eafily be diftinguifhed from the common or working bees. They are both larger and longer in the body. Their heads are round, their eyes full, and their tongues fhort. The form of the belly differs from thofe of both Queen and common bees; and their colour is darker than either. They have no fting, and they make a much greater noife when flying, than either the Queen or the common bees;—a peculiarity of itfelf fufficient to diftinguifh them.

I 2   The

The drones are, by almoſt all writers reckoned the males, (See p. 62,) and are ſo ſtiled by
moſt authors ; but for my part I neither know
what to call them, nor of what uſe they are;
although I have often thought upon the ſubject, yet I cannot be ſatisfied with any theory
I ever heard of. Various conjectures have
been made with reſpect to their uſe. Although
almoſt all agree that they are the males, and
couple with the Queen ; yet they acknowledge
that they never ſaw an inſtance of any one of them
in the act with her. It is ſurely wonderful, if
the drones are the males, that they ſhould have
eſcaped the prying eyes of philoſophers in all
ages, whereas, almoſt every eye has detected
ſmaller inſects in the act.

Swammerdam, ſenſible of this, to ſhelter
himſelf, flies to that falſe refuge, that the *ſmell*
of the drones anſwers the ſame end as copula-
tion. Others ſay, that their heat is neceſſary
for hatching the young bees. But this argument has no weight with me ; as bee-hives
have moſt part of their bees bred, and are well
nigh ſwarming, before any number of drones
appear in the hive. Beſides, by the time that
they become numerous, ſo as their heat might
do good in that reſpect, the heat is generally

ſo

fo great, that the bees have too much of it; and, therefore, often ly out in the fore part of their hive to get air. It is therefore plain, that they need not be at the expence of maintaining a parcel of idle gluttons, for the fake of increaſing what would do them more harm than good.

That the Queen ſtands in no need of their aſſiſtance to fecundate or impregnate her, has already been obſerved, and appears plain, from this conſideration, that ſhe lays eggs, which produce young bees, without having had any previous communication with the drones. I will not, however, ſuppoſe that the drones are of no uſe in the hive; but that the Queen lays eggs which produce young bees, without ſo much as ſeeing a drone; I can with the utmoſt confidence affirm.

The advocates for the old doctrine, that the drones are males, alledge, that they impregnate the Queen, before their brethren kill them. According to this theory, ſhe ſhould continue for no leſs a period than ſeven or eight months, with about 12,000 impregnated eggs in her ovarium, which would certainly make her appear very large during the whole of that period. But it is unneceſſary to waſte

arguments

arguments in refutation of this doctrine, as I have already shown (pages 56, 57, 58) that I have repeatedly had Queens breed and lay eggs, and those eggs become bees, although these Queens were bred seven months after all the drones were dead, and some weeks before any new ones were hatched. These experiments, I think, are sufficient to silence all the arguments advanced by the advocates for the drone system. Mr Debraw, indeed, creates *little drones*, and gives them power to live all the year, and to impregnate the Queen at pleasure. But as room does not permit me to narrate the experiments whereby 1 e attempts to prove this, I shall content myself with stating his sentiments in as few words as possible. He asserts, that, besides the common large drones, which every person, acquainted with bees, knows at first sight, there is a small kind of drones, which are, to all appearance, like the common bees, there being no visible difference, except that they have no sting, which he discovered by immersion in water, and pressure. After relating an experiment on this head, he says, " I once more " immersed all the bees" (of a small swarm) " in water, and when they appeared to be in " a senseless state, I gently pressed every one of
" them

" them between my fingers, in order to diftin-
" guifh thofe armed with ftings from thofe
" that had none, which laft I might fufpect to
" be males. Of thefe I found fifty feven,
" exactly of the fize of common bees, yielding
" a little whitifh liquor on being preffed be-
" tween the fingers."

He farther alledges, that if there be only a
Queen and bees that have ftings in a hive, although the Queen lays eggs, yet if fhe has no
drones to inject the feminal matter upon them,
the eggs will ftill remain unproductive, and
will decay, even although there were 1000 bees
with ftings in the hive. In anfwer to this, I
fhall here narrate an experiment I made feveral years ago.

On the firft of Sept. 1788, I took all the
bees out of a hive that was breeding very faft,
and in which I found only four drones, which
I killed. I put the bees into a hive that had
nothing in it but empty combs. After waiting ten days, upon looking between the combs,
I found maggots newly fealed up, in the cells.
I then took out all the bees, and fhook them into a tub full of water, from which immerfion
I recovered them gradually, and while doing
this, I preffed each bee individually, to try if

I

I could difcover any of thofe ftinglefs little drones ; but not one appeared, all of them having ftings, to the number af 3000. After this I fearched the old hive I had taken them out of, and cut out all the combs that had eggs or young in them ; among which I found fome cells that had new laid eggs in them ; others whofe eggs were converted into a fmall worm, and others fome with maggots in them. I then reftored the Queen, and all the bees, putting them into the fame hive again, but without leaving a fingle egg in it. During the fucceding twenty days, I infpected the hive, and found the bees, in fine weather, working with great alacrity, a fure fign that the Queen was breeding again. After this, on turning up the hive, and cutting out one of the brood combs, I found new laid eggs in fome of them ; others containing maggots ; befides fome young bees, almoft ready to emerge from their cells.

I made another experiment, about the fame time, upon a hive that had fome brood combs, but had not had a large drone for feveral weeks preceding. This hive did not contain above 500 bees, a circumftance that was in my favour, as, being lefs numerous, the trouble was proportionally lefs. I carried the hive into a clofe

room

room in my houfe, that not a fingle bee might efcape me; but, after repeating the former experiment of immerfing them in water, recovering, and preffing them one by one, I found that every one of them had a fting.

I think thefe experiments may fatisfy any unprejudiced perfon, that there is no fuch creature in exiftence as a fmall drone bee; unlefs it be in Mr DEBRAW's *brain*. But, if Mr Debraw, who fays he can find fifty-feven in a fmall fwarm of bees, will fend me the odd feven, I will give him one of my beft hives for them, and I think he will not fay that they are ill fold.

I have often had good hives, with few or no drones in them, during the whole year. Mr KEYS is wrong, when he fays, a top fwarm will not thrive without drones, for I am certain of the contrary. In fummer 1785, I took off four fwarms of my own in one day, without a fingle drone in one of them; yet they all throve well, and the bees bred drones in them about four weeks thereafter.

Although I cannot determine of what ufe the drones are to a hive, unlefs it be to help to confume the honey, which they are very well qualified to do, yet it is obfervable that the

K beft

beſt hives produce them earlieſt in the year;
as they generally appear in ſuch hives about
the beginning of May, and the working bees
put an end to their exiſtence at Lammas, at
which period I generally aſſiſt them as much
as I am able.

After my firſt work upon this ſubjeɑ appeared, I had the honour of a converſation with
two very intelligent gentlemen in my neighbourhood, who declared their ſatisfaɑion with
the arguments I had formerly advanced. I alſo repeated, in the preſence of one of them,
ſome of the ex prmènts I had made, 'to prove
that the common bees are endued with the
power of rearing any egg, from a common cell,
to become a Queen, when the community
ſtands in need of one; and that a Queen, although ſhe never ſaw a drone, will, at a proper
age, lay eggs in abundance, which, again, by
the aſſiſtance of the common bees, will produce
Queens, commons, and drones, as well as thoſe
eggs that are laid by Queens, who are ſur-
rounded with drones in the hives to which
they belong.

After ſeeing theſe experiments, of which he
expreſſed his approbation, I had another converſation with both theſe gentlemen, when
they

they asked me,—What then is the ufe of the
" drone ?"—In anfwer to this, I candidly acknowledged that I could not tell, as any conjecture, that I could form refpecting their ufe,
appeared to be attended with infurmountable
objections. We all agreed, however, that they
certainly muft be of fome ufe, as Nature, or,
more properly fpeaking, the GOD of Nature,
does nothing in vain.

One of the gentlemen faid, that, perhaps
bees might be like fome other infects, whofe
males were not neceffary in every act of generation; and that, perhaps, although a Queen
bee, who had never feen a drone, could lay an
egg which would produce a Queen, and that
Queen again do the fame, and thus the production of Queens and bees be continued with
equal fuccefs, for perhaps fix, eight, or ten generations ; yet it might perhaps turn out, that
thefe Queens would gradually become more
and more unfruitful, and at laft grow altogether barren, unlefs they fhould cohabit with
the drones. The other gentleman, however,
was of opinion, that if one Queen was fruitful without the agency of the drones, every
other one would be fo likewife, to the end of
the world.

K 2   There

There is one thing, however, that feems to favour the former gentleman's conjecture; viz. that fome hives, which had not a fingle drone in them, have been known to breed well for one fummer, pretty well the next, and even tolerably the third; but at laft, have breed drones, and thereby turned out much more prolific thereafter: although it muft be owned, that fuch hives generally fail at laft. Seeing the drones are great confumers of honey, though they do nothing to provide any, fhould the above conjecture, therefore, turn out to be true, a practical inference may naturally be drawn, that a hive may thrive fully as well, or rather better, for 3 or 4 years, without drones than with them; after which period, they might again be introduced into the hive, for the purpofe of renewing the prolific powers of the Queen, and prevent the royal race from becoming barren or extinct. It may be farther obferved, as an additional argument in favour of the above conjecture, that although the Queen and her daughter, none of whom ever faw a drone, might lay abundance of eggs, which would all produce bees; yet they might probably have laid a great many more, had the drones been in the hive with them.

I

I muft confefs, it appears fomewhat paradoxical, to fay that females will breed fuccefsfully for feveral generations without the affiftance of the males ; and yet at laft prove barren, and give over breeding altogether, till their prolific powers are renewed by frefh males cohabitating with them. But however paradoxical or unaccountable it may appear, that is not a fufficient reafon for us to reprobate the fuppofition ; as there are many of the arcana of nature that are equally wonderful and unaccountable, and the elucidation of which has hitherto baffled the inveftigation of the moft penetrating geniufes, and deepeft enquirers into the fecrets of natural philofophy.

One of the above-mentioned gentlemen defired me to try an experiment, and endeavour to afcertain the fact, whether the want of drones will occafion a gradual barrenefs to take place in a fucceffion of Queens. My anfwer was, that I had long entertained an idea of a plan, whereby I am perfuaded that I could dive into, and probably difcover this fecret of Nature ; but that the execution would both require time, and be attended with a confiderable degree of expence, by the lofs of many hives, which at prefent I do not find myfelf
inclined

inclined to rifk.   Whereupon he defired me to
make the experiment with his own hives, which
I engaged to do the firft leifure opportunity :
And as it may doubtlefs be a piece of ufeful
natural philofophy, I fhall certainly communicate the refult of my inquiries to the public
on a future occafion.

CHAP. IX.

ACCOUNT OF THE WORKING BEE.

THE WORKING, or COMMON BEES, are fo often feen by every body, and fo univerfally well
known, that a particular defcription may almoft appear unneceffary, although, for unifor-
mity's fake, I fhall give it.   They are fmaller
in fize than either the Queen or the drone bees ;
and, the denomination they have fo juftly obtained, of *Working* Bees, plainly denotes their
fuperior induftry, in labouring for the whole
hive.

The

The common bee as well as the other two species of that valuable insect, consists of three parts, viz. the head, which is attached by a narrow kind of neck, to the rest of the body;—the breast, or middle part;—and the belly, which is nearly separated from the breast by an insection or division, and connected with it by another narrow neck or junction. There are two eyes in the head, of an oblong figure, black, transparent, and immovable. The mouth or jaws, like those of some species of fish, open to the right and left, and serve instead of hands, to carry out of the hive whatever encumbers or offends them. In the mouth there is a long proboscis, or trunk, with which the bees suck up the sweets from the flowers. They have four wings fastened to their middle part, by which they are not only enabled to fly with heavy loads, but also to make those well known sounds and hummings, to each other, that are supposed to be their only form of speech. They have also six legs fastened to their middle. The two foremost of these are the shortest, and with these they unload themselves of their treasures. The two in the middle are somewhat longer; and the two last are the longest of all. On the outside

of the middle joint of thefe laft, there is a fmall
cavity in the form of a marrow fpoon, in which
the bees collect, by degrees, thofe loads of wax
they carry home to their hives. This hollow
grove is peculiar to the working bee. Neither
the Queen nor the drones have any refem-
blance of it.

The belly is ornamented or diftinguifhed
with fix rings ; and contains, befides the inteftines of the animal, the honey bladder, the venom bladder, and the fting. The honey bladder is a refervoir, into which is depofited the
honey that the bee fips from the cups of the
flowers, after it has paffed through the probofcis, and through the narrow pipes, that con-
nect the head, breaft and belly of the bee.
This bladder, when full, is of the fize of a
fmall pea, and is fo tranfparent, that the colour
of the honey can be diftinguifhed through it.
The fting is fituated at the extremity of the
belly, and the head or root of it is placed con-
tiguous to the fmall bladder that contains the
venom. It is connected to the belly by certain fmall mufcles, by means of which the bee
can dart it out, and draw it in, with great force
and quicknefs. In length it is about the 6th
part of an inch. It is of a horny fubftance ;

is

is biggeft at the root, and tapers gradually towards the point, which is extremely fmall and fharp; and when examined by the microfcope, appears to be polifhed exceedingly fmooth.*. It is hollow within, like a tube, that the venomous liquor may pafs through it, when it ftrikes any animal, which it does the very inftant that the fting pierces the fkin, and infinuates itfelf into the wound; which proves mortal to many fmall animals, as well as to the bee herfelf, when fhe leaves her fting in the wound; as it draws after it the bladder, and fometimes part of the entrails of the bee.

Thefe working bees may be faid to compofe the whole community, except in the feafon of the drones, which hardly lafts three months. During all the other nine months, there are no other bees in the hive, except them and the Queen. The whole labour of the hive is performed by them. They build the combs, collect the honey, bring it home, and ftore it up in their waxen magazines. They rear up the eggs, to produce young Queens, common bees and drones; they carry out all incumbrances that are in the hives; they defend the community againft enemies of every kind, and kill all the drones.

L.   CHAP.

CHAP. X.

DIRECTIONS TO GUARD AGAINST THE STING OF A BEE, WITH THE METHOD OF CURE.

As we muft now proceed to the handling of our induftrious infects, it is neceffary to put our readers on their guard againft their ftings.

Unlefs they are hurt, provoked, or affronted, bees feldom make ufe of their ftings ; but they are fo extremely irritable, that whoever wifhes to be on a friendly footing with them muft beware of giving them the fmalleft offence. They will hazard their lives, rather than let an affront pafs unrevenged ; and, when exafperated near their hives, one may as well take a lion by the beard, or a bear by the fnout, and expect to come off unpunifhed, as to hope to capitulate with them.

When a perfon has any thing to do about his bees, which, he thinks, may provoke their vengeance, and which, neverthelefs, muft be done, fuch as making them fwarm, uniting light hives, &c. then he muft equip himfelf

properly

properly, by putting on his harnefs, * and keeping it on, as long as their rage continues. But
when they are furprifed or frightened by rapping on the hive, they will be very pacific,
and will not attempt to fting. After which,
the Bee-mafter may fafely throw off his harnefs, and even his coat, by which he will be
more fit for performing bufinefs with them.

But fhould they be greatly enraged, the
beft method, if there is a houfe or open door
near, is to run as quickly as poffible into it,
and fhut them out, (for it is eafy to out-run
them,) and thus prevent them from following.
In fuch a cafe they will fly about the door for
fome time in great rage, impatient for an opening

L 2   to

* The HARNESS, or SAFEGUARD, fhould be formed on this plan.
Let a net be knit with fuch fmall mefhes, that a bee cannot pafs
through. Silk, gauze, catgut, crape, or any thing woven of a
fine thread, will anfwer equally well. The fafeguard muft be
made large enough to cover a man's hat, head, and neck, and to
tie clofe together before his breaft with a ftring. In tying it,
great caution fhould be obferved, that not the fmalleft chink or
opening be left for a bee to get in at; otherwife the remedy
will prove worfe than the difeafe; as thofe that get in would fting
with the utmoft virulence, and it would be impoffible to get either the ftings or the bees quickly out from under the harnefs.
The hands fhould be covered with a pair of gloves, and the legs
with a pair of coarfe ftockings, or two pairs of fine ones, as the
bees will often fting the legs through one pair.

to get in ; but the perfon muft take care to remain clofe prifoner, till his winged enemies retire. But if there be no houfe of refuge at
hand, where he can retire by rapid flight, he
fhould by no means retire gradually, but rather ftand ftill like a ftatue, or ly down flat upon
the ground, without any motion, with his face
downwards, in which cafe he may get off with
only two or three ftings ; but if he attempts to
fly and the bees overtake him, they will fting
him in fo many parts at once, that he may
not come off with lefs than one or two dozen
of wounds.

After their fury is abated, and the remem-
brance of the affront entirely obliterated, the
bee-mafter may then renew his acquaintance with his winged labourers ; and if he
comes in a humble manner, and walks gently and fubmiffively among them, they will
treat him kindly. In every bufinefs one has
to do with bees, he muft do it in a calm,
foft, gentle, and fubmiffive way ; he muft
take care not to approach them in a rafh, hafty
manner, puffing and blowing, or accompanied
with any thing that has a difagreeable or un-
favoury fmell, as their organs of fmelling appear to be very acute. In a word, gentle reader,

er, you muſt approach your bees, as you would appear before your patron, when you are going to aſk a favour of him; and not, as you would meet an opponent in a duel, unleſs you be armed cap-a-pee.

When the bees attack a perſon who is walking among them, let him put them gently aſide from his face with his hand, or thruſt his head into a buſh, and they will ſoon leave him.

When they are offended at any perſon, the chief parts they aim at are the face and hands, knowing theſe parts are moſt vulnerable. But if the face and hands are covered, they will ſurround him, and try to diſcover any aperture in his ſhirt, neck, breaſt, ſleeves, breeches-knees, &c. and if they find an opening at the ſmalleſt ſlit or crevice, they will puſh in at it, and leave their ſtings, with their venom behind, though they loſe their lives in the conflict.

The hair of the head, beard, and eye-brows, are all very offenſive to bees, and if they accidentally light on any of them, they will ſting that very inſtant. When at work in the field, they never offer to ſting, let them be ever ſo much affronted. One may then chaſe them

from

from flower to flower, without provoking them
to fting : they rather, on fuch occafions, fly off
from the intruder, as unworthy of their notice.

The ftings of bees have very different effects
on different perfons. There are fome perfons,
upon whom the fting of a bee produces neither inflammation nor pain. Such people need ufe
no precaution, even when they are fure to receive many ftings. Upon others, again, the
fting of a bee, occafions fuch exquifite pain,
accompanied with fwelling and inflammation,
that nothing can terrify them more than the
fight of a bee. This laft clafs fhould not be
difcouraged. I myfelf have felt very different effects from their ftings at different times.
The feldomer I am ftung, and the longer interval that occurs fince 1 was laft wounded,
the greater pain I feel, and the more I fwell :
but when I am ftung twice or thrice in a day,
I value it not a pin. I have fometimes received forty ftings in a day without fwelling
in the leaft. The reafon of this I prefume not
to account for ; I only mention the fact, leaving it to medical people, or thofe who have
ftudied the nature of animal poifons, to inveftigate the caufe.

Many

Many remedies have been prescribed, most of them to little purpose, to cure the wound received by a sting. Oil of olives, or any mild oil, is thought by many to be effectual. Bruised parsley is recommended by others ; the honey taken out of the bee that inflicted the wound, is prescribed by a third class. Some say, that the sweet spirit of vitriol, well rubbed into the wound, will prevent both the pain and the swelling. Repeated experiments, however, have shown that the ease, received from any of the above medicines, is not always to be depended upon, and therefore may be imputed as much to accidental circumstances, such as the wounded person's state of health, blood, &c. as to any peculiar specific virtue; although I doubt not, but that any or all of them may sometimes afford relief.

The sting and its poison are injected in a moment, and the pain and swelling instantly succeed, when such remedies are often very distant. My remedies are more simple, and one or other of them is always at hand. The moment I am wounded, after pulling out the sting, I take a blade of kail, dock, ash, or almost any green leaf of any plant or shrub nearest me, and, bruising it a little, rub the

juice

juice into the wound. When near water, I
wafh the wound, or apply a wet cloth, which
I have fometimes found give relief. But, indeed, I do not, once in a dozen of inftances,
apply any remedy at all, except pulling out the
fting, as it feldom makes me uneafy; and I
know a fhort time and a little patience will
afford an infallible cure.

CHAP. XI.

HOW TO CHOOSE STOCK HIVES IN SEPTEMBER.

ANY perfon, who intends to erect an apiary,
muft take particular care to have it filled with
proper inhabitants. He muft be peculiarly
attentive to this, as all his future profit and
pleafure, or lofs and vexation, will, in general, depend upon it. He muft therefore pay
the utmoft attention to the choice of his ftock
hives; for the man who takes care to keep
good ftock hives will foon gain confiderably
by them; but he who keeps bad ones, will, befides

fides a great deal of trouble, and little or no
fuccefs, foon become a broken Bee-mafter.

In September every ftock hive ought to contain as much honey, as will fupply the bees
with food, till June following; and as many
bees as will preferve heat in the hive, and
thereby refift the feverity of a cold winter, and
act as fo many valiant foldiers, to defend the
community from the invafions of foreign enemies in fpring. And, as September may be faid
to be the bee-mafter's feed time, as well as his
harveft, we fhall begin with it, and go round
the circle of the year, giving fuch directions
as are neceffary to be obferved in the different
feafons, till we arrive again at the fame period.
Therefore the bee-mafter fhould purchafe a
proper number of hives in Auguft, or September, when they are at the cheapeft rate.
They fhould be full of combs, and well ftored
with bees and honey; and fhould weigh at
leaft 30lb. each; if heavier, fo much the better; for light hives run a great rifk of perifhing by famine, unlefs the bees are fupplied
with food; which will coft as much expence,
and a great deal more trouble, * befides a con-

M   fiderable

* However; when a fufficient number of good fingle hives
for

fiderable rifk of their dying at laft, after all this extraordinary trouble and expence. Whereas, a well chofen hive of 30lb. weight, allowing 12lb. for the empty hive, bees, combs, &c. will contain 18lb. of honey, which will fupply the bees with food till next June ; a time, when, it may be prefumed, they will find abundance of provifions for themfelves among the flowers.

When a choice can be obtained, the youngeft hives fhould always be preferred, becaufe old hives are liable to vermin, and other accidents. But although a hive fhould be four or five years old, it fhould not be rejected, if it poffeffes thefe two effential qualities, plenty of bees, and abundance of honey ; but, if either

for ftock cannot be obtained, they may be made up, by conjoining the bees and honey of two or three light hives into one, and thereby making one tolerably good hive out of feveral bad ones. The method of doing this fhall be noticed afterwards ; but it is a meafure that ought never to be adopted but in cafes of neceffity. For neither fuch conjunctions of light hives, nor feeding of bees ought to be adopted, at this feafon, on purpofe to make them ftand the winter's cold, if they can poffibly be avoided. Indeed, fometimes very light hives, with few bees in them, will ftand through the courfe of a mild winter, and do well the following fummer ; but fuch hives are at beft precarious, and therefore not to be depended upon.

either of thefe be a-wanting, the purchafer will regret his bad bargain when it is too late.

C H A P. XII.

OF THE REMOVING OF BEE-HIVES.

I N the removal of hives, the diftance, to which they are to be removed, muft be chiefly, confidered. If it is fmall, they may be tranfported in a hand barrow, carried by two men;—or they may be carried on a man's or woman's head, in the manner that a milk-maid carries her pails.

To prevent the bees from coming out during the carriage, a little ftraw or grafs may be put into the mouth of the hives. But, in warm weather, the greateft care muft be taken, not to fuffocate them with too much heat; efpecially if there is a great number of bees in the hive. For this purpofe, they muft not be fo clofely fhut up, as not to admit abun-

dance

dance of frefh air. For, the great heat of the bees, when no air is admitted, will melt the combs and the honey, and fuffocate or drown the bees, In this manner, valuable hives have often been loft in the fummer feafon, by ignorant perfons, who had been employed to tranfport them, fhutting up the door of the hive fo clofe, that no air could get in. The proper method to prevent the bees from coming out of the hive, in cafe of removal, in warm weather, or indeed at any time, and at the fame time to admit a circulation of air, is, to get a piece of lead or tin plate, pierced full of fmall holes, and fixed to the entry of the hive, This will anfwer both purpofes, by admitting frefh air, and at the fame time preventing the bees from flying away.

When the diftance is great, and there is a confiderable number of hives to be tranfported, (perhaps to the diftance of 6, 12, 20 or 50, miles) into an in-land country, carriages that move on fprings are by all means to be preferred. When thefe cannot be obtained, the hives may eafily be carried on carts or waggons, in cold weather, by placing them with their bottoms upmoft on large quantities of ftraw, hay, or any other foft article. By this method I have

carried

carried 20 hives at one time, with very little damage, either to the bees or the combs. Great care muft be taken in placing them in the cart or waggon, that one hive may not interrupt or intercept the current of air from another. In hot fultry weather, the removal fhould be made in the night.

Before placing the hives in the carriages, every one of them fhould be lifted off the ftool it ufually ftands on, and placed upon a piece of cloth about three feet fquare. This cloth fhould be of the fame texture, with thofe kinds of which window blinds, or cheefe-cloths are made, that it may admit air, at the fame time, that it effectually prevents the bees from efcaping out of the hives. Let it be drawn clofe up, around the edges of the hive, and, when properly fecured to it with pack-thread, not a fingle bee will get out. All this fhould be done the evening before they are removed.

The utmoft care fhould alfo be taken, that no other opening be left at any other part of the hive, for the bees to get out at, as the moft dangerous confequences might arife, as the jolting of the vehicle might provoke the bees to fting both the driver and the horfes; which might occafion the overturning of the carriage, and

and of courfe not only rifk the deftruction of
the whole cargo, with the carriage and horfes,
but even.the life of the driver himfelf.

Another method, if the diftance is great, I
would recommend as preferable to every other,
where it can be obtained, viz. carriage on fhip-
board, either by fea, canals, lakes, or naviga-
ble rivers. By this mode of conveyance, the
bees run no rifk of being jolted or hurt in
the leaft, provided they are properly ftowed in
the veffel. This laft winter, (1794,—5,) I
carried twenty hives on fhip-board, with great
fafety, to a gentleman about 300 miles diftant.
I would, therefore, earneftly recommend water carriage wherever it is practicable, as preferable to every other mode of conveyance
whatever; for I would rather carry a number
of bee-hives 4000 miles by fea, than 100 miles
by land carriage.

CHAP

CHAP. XIII.

HOW TO PREPARE STOCK HIVES FOR WINTER.

AFTER the hives are brought home, if room will permit, let every hive be placed two or three yards afunder, that the bees of one hive may not interfere with thofe of another, as is fometimes the cafe, when the hives are feated near one another, or upon the fame ftandard; for the bees, miftaking their own hives, alight fometimes at the wrong door, and a battle enfues, wherein one or more may lofe their lives. There fhould not be too many hives in one place. Eight or nine are fufficient for one garden*; and as many more may be placed
at.

---

* When too many hives are placed in one apiary, they are often troublefome in fwarming time, by the fwarms going together, and by robbing one another, which they often do in Spring and Autumn, as will be fhown afterwards. Befides, when one has to feed them, the fmell of the honey entices them to fteal from each other, which fometimes occafions many battles, whereby many of the bees are killed. But when there are
not

at about half a mile's diftance in every direc-
tion; and thus the whole kingdom, or even the
whole ifland, might be covered with bee-hives,
at proper regular diftances, wherever there is
a fufficiency of food for the bees to work on.

The hives fhould be placed on boards or ftools,
made of well feafoned wood. Thefe boards fhould
be made a little broader than the bottom of the
hives, and fhould project about fix inches before the entry to it, that the bees may have a
fufficient breadth to alight upon, when they return from the fields. When a proper place is
fixed on, where the hive is to be erected, let
three ftakes be driven into the ground, till the
tops of them are within ten inches of it, and the
foremoft ftake one inch lower than the other
two. The ftool with the hive on it may then
be placed upon thefe; and at fun-fet, let the
fkirts of the hive be plaftered all clofe to the
board with plafter lime. Next, let two fmall
holes be cut, in the under fide of a fmall piece
of hard wood, which muft be fixed to the entry
of the hive with lime. Thefe holes muft juft
be

not too many hives in one place, they are not under fo much temp-
tation to enter into fuch conflicts. But at the fame time, twenty or thirty may be placed in one large apiary, and all do very
well, although the other method is rather to be preferred.

be wide enough to admit the largeſt bee, but no wider, leſt the mice ſhould go into the hive through them †. Each hole ſhould ſcarce exceed a quarter of an inch in heighth and in wideneſs. This ſize muſt be exactly attended to. The whole hive ſhould then be covered all over with a large quantity of pob tow, or ſtraw, which may be fixed to the hive with ropes made of ſtraw, or hay. A large *divot*, or turf, ſhould be laid upon the top of the tow or ſtraw, to hold it cloſe down to the hive, and keep the bees dry and warm. Afterwards, ſome of the

N

tow

---

† Mice are moſt pernicious enemies to bees; for when they get into a hive, they not only eat the honey, but the combs and eggs, and even the bees themſelves. I am perſuaded there are hundreds of hives deſtroyed every year in Britain by theſe vermin. I myſelf, in my younger years, had no fewer than five hives ruined in one winter by theſe rapacious invaders : but now, by taking care to have the entries to my hives made no larger than will juſt admit the largeſt bee, my hives are proof againſt their depredations, and I never loſe either a ſingle bee or a particle of honey by them. The only chance the mice have, when this precaution is obſerved, is to gnaw through the hive itſelf, which they will ſometimes attempt ; but in this they may eaſily be detected and defeated, by taking off the covering now and then.

During the cold months, ſmall ſnails often creep into the hives, and lurk about the inſides of them, though not among the combs : but I never obſerved that they did much hurt. When the hives are turned up in winter to diſcover their ſtate, it is eaſy to diſlodge them, and large ſnails cannot get into the hives, when the entries are made ſmall.

tow or ftraw, fhould be rolled up about four inches above the entry, which will permit the bees to get in thereat; for the lefs that is un-covered of the hive, the drier and warmer it will be, which fhould be aimed at in all feafons, efpecially in winter.

The beft of all covers for hives, however, that I have yet feen or heard of, are fuch as I ordered a potter to make for me of burnt earth-en ware. They are made in the form of a hive, pretty ftrong, about 21 inches wide, and 12 deep; with a circular edging turned up at the fkirts, and a fpout about an inch in length. Thefe, being placed above the pob tow, or ftraw, keep it clofe to the hive, and may eafily be tak-en off or put on at pleafure. The fpout be-ing placed behind, all the water runs off at the back of the hive. The hives, when thus co-vered, may be compared to a man's head with a wig and hat upon it; the pob tow refembling the wig, and the earthen cover the hat. The only objection to thefe covers is, that they are brittle, and eafily broken; but the care, that every good bee-mafter will readily beftow upon his hives in any cafe, is fufficient to preferve them from accidents of this kind. I fold a-bove 30 of thefe covers to a gentleman in Northumberland

thumberland about three years ago, and I have reafon to believe that there is not one of them yet broken.

CHAP. XIV.

HOW TO MANAGE BEES IN WINTER.

THE hives in September, being properly placed, covered, and made fit to endure the winter, there is very little more neceffary to be done, for about three months. This feafon may, therefore, be called *the Bee-mafter's refting time.* It will be proper, however, occafionally to take care, that the covers continue to ftand firmly upon the hives, and that no mice neftle about them. When the froft is fevere, or when fnow is lying on the ground, it will be neceffary to prevent the bees from coming out of the hives, by fhutting up their entry quite clofe with pobtow; which will keep them warm, at the fame time that they will run no rifk of fuffocation in

　　　　　　　　　very

very cold weather.* In extreme colds, the hives
may be taken into out-houfes, which will preferve

* Bees fhould by no means be difturbed in cold weather, fo
as to provoke them to go abroad out of their hives, unlefs fome
very important object is in view: For, not only in winter, but
even in fpring, fummer and autumn, if they fly out of their hives
in cold or wet days, efpecially in the evenings or mornings, and
alight on the ground, their active powers become inftantly fo
benumbed, that often within half a minute thereafter, they
will be rendered totally unable to rife, in confequence of
which they muft crawl about till they perifh. If bees are permitted to go abroad in time of fnow, which they are tempted to _
do, by the glare of the light, they will alight upon it, and fip a
little ; but their delicate bodies are foon fo chilled by the cold,
that their wings lofe their power of raifing them, and inevitable
death fucceeds.

Every other part of the hive, as well as the entry, fhould be
carefully examined, to difcover if it be all quite clofe ; for after
long confinement, efpecially when the feafon is advanced to a-
bout the middle of February, the bees will make every poffible
attempt to get out of the hive, as their own ordure then becomes
offenfive to them. At times, when I have thought the entry to
the hive was made fo completely fecure, that not a fingle bee
could get out at any opening. yet, in walking through my apiary,
I have difcovered them making their way through places, where
I could not have fuppofed they would have attempted an efcape.
When bees are completely fhut up in a good clofe hive, they are
in a ftate of perfect darknefs ; but, if there be the fmalleft aperture in any part of it, the light, fhining through it, leads them
directly to the place ; when they are apt to make every poffible
effort to widen it, and, in fuch cafes, they will often fqueeze
through

ferve them from cold. But, indeed, when the hives are properly covered, and the entries to them clofely ſhut up, they will refiſt a very ſevere cold.

Many ingenious gentlemen have tried different methods to preſerve bees in winter. Some have ſhut them up in cold out-houſes, from September to April; others only from the 1ſt of November to March. A third claſs place grates before their entries, to admit air, but keep the bees cloſe in their hives, during the whole winter.

The limits of this performance will not permit me to enlarge upon the fruitleffneſs of theſe inventions. Suffice it therefore to obſerve

through a very narrow hole. It is therefore adviſeable, though the hives may be ſuppoſed perfectly cloſe, to infpect them frequently, left any bees ſhould get out at an unfufpected place, and not only periſh themfelves, but leave an opening for invaders to get in. Befides, upon returning to their hives, they will go to their uſual entry to get in again, and not finding admittance, will wander about in ſearch of it, till they periſh, unleſs they chance to alight upon the aperture by which they had got out. The ſame caution muſt be obſerved, when a hive is ſhut up at any other ſeafon of the year, or upon any account whatever.

I have ſometimes picked up great numbers of wandering bees from off the cold ground, or ſnow, and, after recovering them by gradual warmth, have reſtored them again to their hives,

ferve in general, that long confinement is prejudicial to the health of the bees; and that, as
they do eat a little during their confinement,
it is neceffary that they fhould get out to void
their ordure; for, I have even feen bees, in
fome hives that have been long confined, fwell-
ed to fuch a fize, for want of fuch opportunities, that they feemed larger than a Queen bee;
and, when they did at laft get liberty to go
out of their hives, being unable to fly, they
would fall over the edge of their ftool, and
creep about on the ground, till they died in
great numbers; fo that fcarce one of a dozen
of them ever recovered. But when they are
permitted to go out occafionally, in fine winter days, they get fo much benefit by the free
air, and by eafing their bodies in flying, that,
when they return to their hives, they are able
to turn out the dead bees, and they conclude
the day with a *fong*;—a fure fign that they are
healthy and happy. In fhort, I find by experience, that bees thrive beft, when the hives
are allowed to ftand out, and when the bees
are at liberty to go out and in at pleafure in
fine days, even in winter; for they are wife
enough to know when they may venture out
with fafety; and they will come to the door

of

of their hive to eafe nature, and return again, when the weather forbids their going abroad.

It is faid by many writers on this fubject, that a fine winter is dangerous to the bees, and that many more of them die in a mild winter than in a cold one. They argue, that as the appetite of the bees increafes by their going often out, they confume their provifions, and die of famine; whereas, when long confined in their hives, they hardly eat any. * I acknowledge

* Some Authors, particularly Mr Stephen White, alledge, that fevere cold is rather falutary for bees, as it keeps them in a torpid ftate, in confequence of which they eat none at all. I acknowlege, that they eat much lefs in cold weather than in warm, becaufe they have little or no exercife, and their appetite increafes or decreafes in proportion to the exercife they take. In November, December, and January, bees eat very little food, as any perfon may be convinced, by weighing their hives in the begining and the end of thefe months, when he will find very little difference in point of weight. But if he will weigh a hive in the beginning of March, and weigh it again at the end of it, he will find a confiderable decreafe; for the bees, having now much exercife, eat more honey during that month, than during all the three above mentioned cold months; and I am perfuaded, that they devour three times as much in May as in March, owing to the fame caufe operating in an increafing proportion. But that the bees eat *none at all* in cold weather is a great miftake, and may eafily be refuted: For let any perfon, in winter, put a number of bees into a hive that has nothing but empty combs,
and

knowledge, that, in a mild winter, they do eat
more food than in a cold one, when they cannot get out ; but this, as well as the fine air,
contributes greatly to their health ; besides that
they hatch earlier, and confequently increafe
the number of bees in the hives fooner. The
fact is, that experience, which is preferable to
the conjectural reafoning of the moft eminent
authors, may convince any perfon, that many
more bees die in fevere winters than in mild
ones. In winter 1776 which was very cold,
a great number of Bee-hives perifhed ; and alfo
during laft winter, (1794-5) being an exceffive-
ly

and let them be kept equally cold with thofe in hives that contain both honey and bees, and a trial of eight or ten days will
convince him, that *honey*, and not *cold*, is the proper food of
bees.

In the very midft of a fevere froft, I have often feen my hives
with young broods in them ; a fure fign, that they were neither motionlefs, nor in a ftate of inactivity. This fact alfo proves
how greatly miftaken many authors are, who affert, that bees do
not breed, till they begin to carry home loads in fpring. I am
confident, that there is not a month in the whole year, in which
I have not feen many of my hives, with fome eggs as well as
young bees in the cells ; although there are at leaft four months
in the year in which the bees carry home no loads. I will allow, however, that although they do breed fome in winter, the
number is very fmall. Perhaps the Queen does not lay above
three or four eggs in a day, whereas in fummer fhe will lay daily
above a hundred.

ly fevere one, many hives were deftroyed from that caufe alone; whereas in winter 1779, which was remarkably mild, not one hive in twenty failed; and the bees, in general, fwarmed a month earlier than ufual.*

I have feen the bees of a hive that had been long confined by cold, (perhaps for ten weeks,)

O   fo

* Mr Wildman fays, page 249, " The degree of cold, which " bees can endure has not been afcertained. We find that they " live in the cold parts of Ruffia, and often in hollow-trees, " without any care being taken of them." Page 252, he fays, " that bees fuffer fuch degrees of cold, as we here are ftrangers " to, without detriment, feems certain; nor is it eafily accounted " for, why a much lefs degree of cold becomes fatal to them " in our mild climate. If I may venture my opinion, I think " that in thefe extreme colds, the bees are fo perfectly frozen, " that their juices cannot corrupt or putrify but they remain in the " fame ftate till the return of fpring; when the change of the " weather being fudden, the bees foon come to life; whereas in " our climate they are fo far chilled as to lofe the figns of life, " and their juices being ftill in a liquid ftate, foon putrify, and " real death enfues with corruption."

With all due deference, I fhall now venture to give my opinion, on this point. I would account for it in this manner; that the fame *degree* of cold will prove equally fatal to bees in Britain, Russia, Siberia, or any other place in the world; and that whenever the cold is fo great, as to render the bees entirely *motionlefs*, they will continue in that ftate for ever; or, in other words, they will *die*; unlefs they be recovered by heat,

before

fo difeafed, that, when good weather returned, and they came abroad, very great numbers would have died within a day or two thereafter; and the hive in general would have been greatly reduced. It is evident, that their long confinement

before putrifaction takes place, which will otherwife happen within two days at moft, after they are frozen. Laft winter (1794-5) it was perhaps as cold here, at leaft for one week during the ftorm, as it is in Ruffia or Siberia, in fome moderate winters. Some of our bees were, at that period, as completely and irrecoverably frozen, during thofe eight days, as ever any hive could be in Ruffia; and all the heat that human power could apply, however gradual or moderate, could not have recovered them to life again.

As a proof of this, any perfon may make the following experiment: Take a bee, during a hard froft, and lay it upon a ftone; within two minutes it will be frozen, and to all appearance dead. If it ly on the ftone, for fix or eight hours, it will be as completely frozen, as if it had been eight days in the coldeft place in the world. Yet, by warming it in a warm bed, for half an hour, it may be brought to life again; whereas, if it be allowed to ly for eight days upon the fame ftone, (during which time it would be as completely frozen, as if it had been eight days in Ruffia) neither the heat of a bed, nor any other degree of heat whatever, will ever be able to recover it. On the whole, I am of opinion, that all poffible care fhould be taken to preferve bees from fevere cold in every corner of the world; and I doubt much, if ever there was a fingle hive, that was once completely frozen for twenty days, that, even in Ruffia itfelf, or any other part of the globe, was ever recovered to life again.

confinement was the caufe ; but it is alfo certain, that, even in thofe cold countries, where
the winter lafts eight months, bees thrive and
profper well, elfe they never could produce fo
much honey*. I have known bees do well, however, that had been confined in their hives for
five months, even in this country ; while o-
thers of them were ready to perifh, by retain-
ing their fœces for fo long a period. Sometimes, about Martinmas, I have feen four hives,
ftanding in one place, all equally thriving and
numerous ; but, in confequence of having been
confined by bad weather for fix or eight weeks
after that period, one of thefe hives would have
had feveral hundreds of dead bees, lying fwoln
on the ftool, while the other three were ftill in
a thriving condition, and had fcarcely a dozen
dead bees in each. Upon tearing one of the
dead bees afunder, I found her inteftines quite
full of fœces ; which, I therefore conjectured,

was

---

* The reafon may be acounted for in this manner ; fuppofe, for
inftance, that one fourth part of the bees in thofe places fhould
fail by long confinement or fevere colds, (from which I fuppofe
the natives will guard their bees as much as poffible,) yet the
remaining three parts will increafe greatly in bees and honey during their fummer, as the weather is very conftant and warm
while the honey feafon lafts.

was the caufe of her death; whereas the inteſ-
tines of the thriving bees had very little matter in them, and therefore, I am inclined to
think that this was the reafon of their continuing healthy and active. Whether the original difeafe of the former clafs, and their pre-
mature deaths, proceeded from their gluttony,
in gormandizing more food than was neceſſary; or whether it was an epidemical difeafe
that had got in among them, and carried them
off in fuch numbers, I will not prefume to determine; though I rather incline to the former
opinion. But, from whatever caufe the difeafe
proceeds, fuch hives often lofe their inhabitants at the rate of a dozen or more *per* day,
till they are greatly reduced, or perhaps quite
defolated at laſt.

For fuch misfortunes, I know of no remedy
or even preventative; but it is fortunate, that
fcarcely one or two hives of a dozen meet
with them. Sometimes I have united the living
bees, that remained of fuch a hive, with thofe
of a healthy one, but feldom found it turn
out well; owing perhaps to this caufe, that the
difeafe was really contagious, and the difeafed
bees might carry the infection along with
them, and thereby hurt the healthy hive. I
generally,

generally, therefore, let the remaining bees of
fuch an unfortunate hive, take their chance;
and on the firſt favourable day allow them to
fly about, and difcharge their burdens, which
muſt doubtlefs enable them to return to the
hive with a greater degree of health; but I am
confident that many of the difeafed ones never
return, and indeed the hive will be fully as
well without them.

About the middle of January, every hive
may be gently lifted off the ſtool, and the
ſtate of it examined. The ſtool ſhould then
be carefully cleanfed of dead bees, or any filth
that may have gathered upon it during the
winter. The hive ſhould then be replaced u-
pon the ſtool, and carefully plaſtered about the
fkirts again, and covered over as formerly. If
the bees of any hive have deferted it, and
gone into another, which they fometimes do,
(as ſhall be further noticed in a fubfequent
chapter,) the hive may be carefully kept, in order to feed bees with the honey it contains in
fpring, or to receive a young fwarm in fummer.

CHAP

CHAP. XV.

DIRECTIONS HOW TO SUPLY BEES WITH FOOD.

As bees fometimes run fhort of provifions, efpecially when there is a long continuance of cold
or wet weather, during Spring, or even in the beginning of Summer, it is abfolutely neceffary to
re-inforce the hives, efpecially the light ones,
with additional ftore. There are four methods
of fupplying the hives in fuch cafes, which I
fhall lay before the reader, and one or other of
which, every bee-mafter fhould attend to, at
fuch feafons of the year as he finds his bees
will need a re-inforcement of provifion.

I. The firft, and indeed the beft method is
by *eeking**. Take an eek,* of fix or eight rows
deep, and place it on a ftool, with the quantity

---

* ** To *eek*, in the Scotch dialect, fignifies literally to *add* to
any thing. The *eek*, or *addition* here meant, is a part of an old
hive, cut down on purpofe, to give room for placing the fupply of
povifion under the deficient hive,

ty of honey, neceffary to 'fupply the deficient
hive, within it, which may be from one to
four, or even eight pounds of honey, according to the deficiency that appears, and the
number of bees in the hive. The combs
fhould be placed in the eek, in fuch a pofition,
that the bees may have free accefs to the honey,
on all fides. At night, let the deficient hive be
gently placed upon the eek, and let the inter-
ftices between the hive and the eek be plaftered up with lime; after which let the entry be
fhut, that neither native bees nor ftrangers
may get accefs. Let the hive and the eek continue in this fituation for 24 hours; in which
time the bees will have removed all the loofe
particles of the honey, and the fmell of it will
not be fo apt to invite ftrange bees. The entry at the bottom of the eek may, therefore,
now be opened, and the bees allowed free e-
grefs and accefs. 'If the additional quantity of
honey given in the eek did not exceed a pound
or two, the eek may be removed within three
or four days; but if it amounted to fix or eight
pounds, it may be allowed to remain for fix
weeks in Spring. ‡ If, in September, a hive
has

* This method may be practifed at all feafons of the year,
and

has got an additional fupply of twelve or fixteen pounds, it fhould be allowed to remain at
leaft as many weeks, if not altogether ; only at
this feafon, place all the combs in the eek, in
the fame order in which they were naturally
in the hive they were taken from ;—the uppermoft cells to be ftill upermoft, and fo of
the reft, leaving a fpace of an inch and a half
between the combs. The combs muft be fixed
with fticks to make them ftand on their edges,
and they fhould run as much in the fame di-
rection as poffible, with thofe in the hive. The
bees will foon join the combs together, and
render them fit to be lifted all at once. In
Spring, if the original hive be large, the eek
and combs may be removed, but if fmall, they
fhould both remain during Summer.

II.

and it has this additional advantage, that it may be executed at
little expence, and occafion a faving of all the honey in the old
combs that will not run out, or that happens to be mixed with
bee-bread, eggs, or young bees. All fuch honey ought to be
thrown into thefe *granaries*, and the bees will foon carry up all
the honey, and place it in their own refervoirs, leaving only the
empty combs, which can be melted and made into wax afterwards. It need hardly be added, that the bees do not, in fuch
cafes, inftantly eat all the additional honey that is given them,
but only lay it up for future ufe.

II. The second method is the fame with the preceding, but differs only in this particular; that when the Bee-mafter has no old combs with honey in them, he muft melt frefh honey, and pour it into large empty combs, of which drone combs are the beft, and place them into the eek as above directed.

III. The third method is, to fave the trouble of eeking the hive, (when a fmall quantity may ferve,) by placing a comb, with melted honey in it, upon the ftool, immediately before the entry of the deficient hive, and leaving it entirely to the induftry of the bees, to collect and carry it into the hive. The only difadvantage of this method is, that ftrange bees will be tempted to moleft the natives, in confequence of which a battle may enfue, and fome lives may be loft. But, to prevent this, let the honey be given at a time of the day when no bees are abroad, and the danger will be avoided. I have fometimes had a dozen of hives in one apiary, with a feeding comb placed before each; which gave all the bees of each hive fo much employment at their own doors, that they had neither time nor inclination to moleft or rob their neighbours.

IV. The fourth method is, to turn up the

P

deficient

deficient hive, and, laying it on one fide, to pour
melted honey into the empty cells, where there
are few or no bees; and, when the one fide of
all the combs are properly filled, to turn up
the other, and fill their empty cells with honey
alfo. A tea-pot is moft proper for executing
this plan. In this manner I have fometimes
poured two pounds of honey into a hive at a
time. When the hive is again placed on the
ftool, a little honey will run down from the
combs upon it; but the entry being clofe fhut
up, will prevent robbers from fmelling the treafure, and will keep fuch bees, as may have been
befmeared with honey during the operation,
within the hive. The native bees will foon
not only lick up all the fpilt honey from the
ftool, but will alfo fuck it off the backs of their
befmeared brethren, and lay it up in their refervoirs, with fo much expedition, that next
day not a drop of it will be vifible, either on
the ftool or on the bodies of the bees.

It is not to be doubted, that, in cafes of necef-
ty, bees may be fed and preferved with other
articles, befides honey; fuch as fugar, fweet
wort, treacle and the like : but I am of opinion,
that they cannot be fed, either at lefs expence
or with as much fafety, with any other thing
than

than their own natural food. To give them any other fubftitute, would occafion as much expence, and a great deal of more trouble, efpecially when the hives are well filled with inhabitants : and I dare venture to fay, that as fuch methods have never yet been much adopted, fo, if ever they fhould, they will not turn out to the proprietors advantage, or become of general ufe, in the prefervation of bees. But it muft be owned, that, if no honey can be obtained to feed bees with, in fpring, fome of the above fubftitutes will fupply the deficiency tolerably well. In fuch a cafe, let 1 lb. of brown fugar be mixed with half a gill, (or half a quartern) of fmall beer, and let a table fpoonful at a time be placed before the entry to the hive, as above recommended in the third method. Let this be repeated daily as long as is neceffary, and the hive will be preferved from famine, and will in all probability do well; but when a hive is light in September, it ought to be fupplied with nothing but honey.

P 2 CHAP.

CHAP. XVI.

OF THE WARS AND ROBBERIES THAT TAKE PLACE AMONG THE BEES.

IT cannot be denied, that the animals, who are the subject of this treatise, have their *vices*, as well as their *virtues*. To the virtues of *industry* and *oeconomy*, which they are endued with in an eminent degree, we must add, what some would call a *martial spirit*, but which rather deserves to be denominated, a spirit of *theiving* and *robbery*. For when the weather is good, and there are not flowers in the fields for the bees to work on, they will risk their lives by robbing other hives, and strive to enrich their own hive at the expence and ruin of their neighbours. In such cases, the hives that are thinly inhabited, are ready to fall a prey to the bold invaders; for hardly one hive within their reach is left unaffaulted; and as, among mankind, the strong overpower and

subjugate

subjugate the weak, so a weak hive sometimes falls a prey to a set of strong invaders; but when strong and *populous* hives (so to speak,) are attacked by a less numerous body of robbers, they give them a terrible reception, and hardly a single bee, that they can get hold of, gets off to tell his neighbours the fate of his brethren. Sometimes a good number of hives will join in robbing one single hive. In such a case, all is confusion and rage, and great slaughter takes place. The bees are seen flying in the air like so many fiery dragons ready to attack every one; and whoever dares obstruct their flight, will feel their poisonous spears in a moment. At such a time, one dare scarcely venture near them, unless he is resolved to receive wounds from all quarters. When they are engaged thus, their sound in the air is easily distinguished.

The people's actions will their thoughts declare,
All their hearts tremble, and beat thick for war.
Hoarse broken sounds, like trumpets harsh alarms,
Run through the hive, and call them forth to arms :
All in a hurry spread their shiv'ring wings,
And fit their claws, and point their angry stings :
In crouds before the hive they all do light,
And boldly challenge out the foe to fight.

VIRGIL.

Various reasons have been assigned for this propensity of the bees to rob one another. A majority of writers impute it to the following causes :

1*st*, The scarcity of provisions : The bees of one hive, finding they have not sufficient provision for themselves, and the season being backward, try to enrich themselves at the expence of their neighbours.

2*dly*, The artificial feeding of hives : When one hive is fed, their neighbours, smelling the fresh honey, wish for a share of it, and will take no denial, though it should cost them their lives : which it often does, the inhabitants of the fed hives standing up most heroically in defence of their property. This consideration will lead the attentive Bee-master to study the utmost caution and prudence in feeding such hives as require extra supplies ; else the remedy will prove worse than the disease.

3*dly*, But the chief reason is, their insatiable avarice for honey.— In spring and autumn, when the weather is good, but little or no honey can be collected from plants, all bees whatsoever are apt to go a *marauding* and plundering their neighbour's hives ; although, it must
be

be owned, the pooreft are moft addicted to pil-
fering.

Here it is neceffary to inform the reader,
how thefe robbers are to be diftinguifhed as
well as how to get rid of them. When a number of bees are feen crowding into a hive, and
many dead bees lying flaughtered before the
gates ;—when others are feen flying as if af-
frighted, and the native bees purfuing, catching, wreftling, and buftling with them upon
the ftool, in a moft furious manner, then it
may be fafely inferred that robbers are attack-
ing the hive; which indeed, if it be weak in
numbers, will not be worth preferving. In
that cafe, the beft way will be, to turn up the
hive, and diflodge the robbers by rapping upon
it, and at night to put the bees belonging to
it into any other hive that will receive them.
The manner of doing this will be taken notice
of, when we come to mention the beft mode of
re-inforcing a hive. But if the hive that is
attacked be tolerably full of valiant bees, who
withftand their foes ftoutly, then let the entry
be made fo fmall, that only one bee can get in
at once, and let fome perfon ftand before the hive
with a light cloth in his hand, to wave the robbers afide, and keep them off, till a fhower of
rain,

rain, or night coming on, or perhaps a dark cloud intercepting the fun's rays, oblige the invaders to retreat. Next morning, if the weather be good, let the hive be shut up close, to prevent the robbers from getting access; and let it continue so for some time, till the invaders give over their attempt; but if they continue their inroads daily, let the hive be removed to the distance of a mile or so; and indeed this is the most effectual method to free the hive from farther molestation.

In my younger years, these robberies gave me much uneasiness, as I was alarmed at the sight of a slaughtered bee; but now I give myself no concern, as I either put the bees of the hive that is attacked into another hive, or remove them to a proper distance from danger. I have frequently, indeed, seen some sore battle take place among my own bees, and last for perhaps a day or two; after which a peace would have ensued, without my interference. But good hives seldom suffer much by robberies; perhaps not one in fifty. They may indeed lose a score of bees or so, but that will never hurt them.

CHAP.

CHAP. XVII.

DIRECTIONS HOW TO MANAGE BEES IN MARCH, APRIL, AND
MAY.

IN spring, hives are sometimes found without
a single bee in them, and the owner, in such
cases, is at a loss to account for the cause.
The following circumstance, which occurred
among my own bees, will throw some light on
this subject.

The long continuance of the late storm
(1794-5) having confined the bees in their
hives for about four months, the bees of some
hives contracted diseases, which, during the
last month of their confinement proved very
fatal to them; and some of them daily fell
down, or rather *came* down of their own accord, from the combs to the stool, in search of
some aperture to get out at, in order to void
their fœces; but, after crawling about on the
bottom of the hive for a considerable time in

Q   vain

vain, the cold benumbed them fo much, that
they could not return to their brethren again,
and thus death enfued. Now, fuppofing only
three dozen of bees *per* day to have come down
upon this errand, and perhaps not a third of
them to have been able to return, it is evident,
that fuch hives muft of courfe be foon greatly
reduced in the number of their inhabitants.
This made me anxious for good weather, that
my difeafed and diftreffed fervants might get
out, and recover their health, by flying about
and getting rid of their fuperfluous matter.
The long wifhed for period at laft arrived.
The ftorm broke, and the weather became
mild ; and, upon examining my hives, I found,
that out of fourteen, which I had in one
apiary, there were twelve whofe bees were in
a healthy ftate ; and that thofe of the remaining two were partly difeafed. The day being
very fine, and the doors of my hives opened,
the bees flew about as thick as hail, making a
great noife with their ufual mufic. My wife
being prefent, we obferved, that the two difeafed hives gradually diminifhed in the number
of their bees, whereupon I faid, that I fuppofed the bees would foon defert thefe hives
altogether ; to which fhe replied, that fhe wifhed

ed

ed they would, and that they would go into
some other hives, provided they did not fight.
Upon farther obfervation, I found, that fome
of them entered into one hive, and fome into
another, till at laft the original hives were totally deferted, except the Queen and about a
fcore of bees; and that almoft all the bees entered into thofe hives that were moft happy,
as appeared by their making a moft harmonious found at the entry of their hives, by which
mufic they feemed to invite and welcome their
new friends. The deferted hives were well
ftored with honey, and therefore I turned
them upfide down, and placed them below
fome of my other hives, in order that the bees
might collect the honey that was in them.
Such deferted hives I have often found ufeful
for putting a young fwarm into.

I have even feen young fwarms gradually
defert their hives in this manner, and go into
other hives. When they go into one of their
own mafter's hives, I never fee any lofs by it,
efpecially when they unite peaceably; as one
good hive is worth four bad ones.

It is worthy of obfervation, that the bees, on
this occafion, deferted the weak hives gradually, and not in a body, as they do when they

fwarm

fwarm ; and alfo, that it may happen at particular times, that different men's bees, ftanding in the fame apiary, or near each other, may
join together.   Therefore, to prevent fuch circumftances from taking place, to the prejudice
of others, it is neceffary to allot a proper diftance between one man's hives and thofe of a-
nother.

Thofe who live in places where vegetation
is generally late, if they take the trouble to remove their hives to more early fituations, efpecially if they have a great number of them,
will foon find themfelves doubly repaid for
their trouble and expence, as their bees will
thereby both breed and fwarm much earlier.
I would indeed advife every bee-mafter, who
conveniently can, to keep two apiaries, an early and a late one, in confequence of which, his
bees will be conftantly employed, when the
weather is favourable, during the whole working feafon.

In fpring I generally fhut up the doors of
my hives every evening, as foon as the bees
are all got in, and open them again next morning ; and I even do this for whole days during
that feafon, when the cold is fevere ; as cold
winds blowing in at their entries are extremely

ly prejudicial to them, and ought therefore to be prevented with all poffible care. By this fimple practice, the bees are kept warm and healthy, which is greatly beneficial to them in breeding. But in following this plan, great caution muft be obferved, that the bees have no other vent to get out at, as the confequences would be fatal. (See pages 100 and 101.)

In the beginning of March, if the weather be good, the bees will begin to carry home loads of honey and wax. I have feldom feen them carry fo early as February, excepting in the year 1793, when I obferved feveral bees go into one of my hives, heavy loaden, fo early as the term of Candlemas; but I believe they hardly carried any more for a full month thereafter.

At this feafon, every hive ought to be again lifted, and the ftool cleaned; on which occafion, the ftate of the hive, both with regard to its provifions, and the number of its inhabitants, will be difcovered. Hives of twenty pounds weight ftand in no need of any fupply of food, and may therefore be immediately replaced upon their ftools, and covered, and their fkirts plaiftered as iormerly; but, fuch as weigh only fourteen or fixteen pounds fhould

be

be reinforced with fix pounds of honey comb, as directed in page 110. Three pounds of honey will be a fufficient fupply for fuch as weigh eighteen pounds. Some hives perhaps will not exceed fourteen pounds or fo; yet, if they have few bees, they will not need to be fupplied; for, befides that they ftand in no need of it, a frefh fupply of honey would invite robbers, whom they would not be able, on account of the paucity of their numbers, to withftand. A thinly inhabited hive ought, therefore, never to be reinforced with honey, unlefs the bees are ready to perifh for want of food, which, in fuch a hive, feldom if ever happens. But a hive that is well peopled ought to be abundantly fupplied, even although there may appear to be a fufficiency of food, becaufe the fuperfluity will not be loft. The bees are faithful ftewards, and will not fail to repay their mafter's generofity with ufury. *

For

* The fupplying of bees with food, in any feafon, but efpecially in fpring, is of great advantage to them, as it cheers their fpirits, and roufes them to breed earlier than they otherwife would. I would therefore recommend to every bee-mafter, to give a little additional food, even to hives that have abundance, in order to revive and exhilarate the bees, and encourage them

to

For I am confident, that when they are fully fed, they will breed faft, even in bad weather; whereas, if they have little provifion of their own, and receive no extra fupply, they will breed very flowly.

From this, as well as from other peculiarities in the nature of thefe infects, it appears pretty evident, that they are endued with a high degree of free or voluntary agency, as they can breed early or late, frequently or feldom, at pleafure, and according to circumftanees. All poffible attention, therefore, fhould be paid to the full feeding of bees in Spring, and alfo in the beginning of fummer, if the weather be unfavourable.

A hive will fometimes lofe their Queen in fpring, and of courfe will go to ruin, as it will then be impoffible for the bees to raife another, if they have not an egg to raife one from. A hive may be known to be in this fad predicament, by the following fymptoms: The bees
will

to hatch their young families, early in the feafon. But fuch hives as weigh heavy in March or April, having plenty of honey, with bees in them carrying well, may be fafely allowed to remain without any frefh fupply of food, as they will profper without it; although, if the owner has time and abundance of honey, he may reap additional profit by giving them a little.

will immediately give over working as foon as
the young in the cells are fealed up; and one
may wait an hour at the hive without feeing a
loaded bee enter it.   The bees then confume
their own honey faft, and an uncommon number of them generally croud about the entry:
And if the hive has been long without a Queen,
upon turning it up, and fearching for maggots
in the cells, they will be found quite empty.

As foon as thefe melancholy figns are obferved, the owner fhould directly take out all the
bees, and unite them with thofe of fome other
hive, that has few bees in it, the manner of
doing which will be afterwards mentioned:
and if the hive be young, it may be kept to
put a young fwarm into, but if old, the honey
fhould be laid afide for ufe.

Sometimes, in fpring, I have found, in particular cells in hives, a confiderable number of
young that, from fome caufe or other, had decayed and never come to perfection, as mentioned, page 64. I have fometimes obferved
the number of thefe fo great, that in one comb,
containing perhaps 600 young bees, the one
half would have been in this ftate in the cells.
The effluvia proceeding from thefe abortive
productions, gave the hive a favour by no
means

means agreeable to me, and which muft doubt
lefs have been very difgufting to the bees. I
have often endeavoured to inveftigate the caufe
of thefe phænomena, but am as yet unable to
fatisfy myfelf, unlefs perhaps it be owing to
extreme cold. But againft this fuppofition the
objection naturally arifes, that fome eggs in the
fame hive, and in the fame degree of cold, produce bees which arrive at full maturity ; and,
therefore, in reply, it muft be taken for granted, that fome eggs are naturally more able to
bear cold than others ; and, indeed, it is moft
commonly in hives that are but thinly inhabited, that fuch misfortunes take place.

To diftinguifh hives in this condition, therefore, the following criterion may ferve. In
fpring, when bees, which formerly carried well,
and ftill are in no want of food, give over carrying, let the hive be directly turned up, and
infpected between the combs. Then, upon taking a fmall ftick, and putting it down among the
thickeft of the bees, where the maggots lie fealed up, and with it rubbing off the tops of two
or three of the fealed cells, if frefh whitifh
maggots appear, it may be concluded, that the
brood is coming forward : but if the cells appear quite empty, or if only blanched maggots

R   appear

appear in a number of them, then it is certain that the brood is going backward.

If such a hive has but few bees, it will be proper to unite them with another hive; but if it has a confiderable number of bees, they fhould be allowed to continue to work on, in the beft way they can, till the beginning of June, when the ftrong hives begin to lay out; at which time a great number of common bees fhould be taken from one or two of them, to re-inforce that hive with, in the manner that fhall be afterwards pointed out. I have feen a hive, with a vaft number of fuch rotten eggs and decayed maggots in it, in April, which, when allowed to remain till June, and being re-inforced with frefh bees, would have turned out a fine thriving hive before autumn; although many of the decayed eggs and maggots would have ftill been in it: For I believe fome fuch abortions may continue in a hive for-years, perhaps with little detriment to the bees; for they in time dry up, and wither away in the cells, and their bad favour gradually goes off. Such hives, however, fhould always be taken in autumn; and their bees united to more thriving hives. *

In

* Formerly I ufed to cut out the combs containing the moft
rotten

In May, if cold, mifty, or cloudy weather, continues for a few days, the bee-mafter fhould pay particular attention to his hives, left any of them fhould be in danger of fa-mine ; for, at this period, the number of bees in each hive is greatly increafed, and of courfe they quickly confume the remains of their winter and fpring provifion, fo that even the very beft of hives will be in danger. When fuch weather occurs, therefore, in May or e-ven in June, let every hive get fome additional food, in order to prevent all danger of fa-mifhing, now that they are juft upon the brink of their honey harveft. For, as foon as the muftard bloffoms, and the white clover appear on the lees, they will make the very air to fmell

R 2   of

rotten eggs, and the moft decayed maggots, whereby I cleared the hive of a great nuifance, which I thought it would be much the better of wanting. But, in doing this, I found that the removal of fuch maffes of combs occafioned a large vacancy in the hive, and thereby made it colder. To remedy this defect, I have fome times put a piece of frefh comb in its place, in which I found the Queen foon laid eggs again. But ftill, as in thefe combs, containing the decayed eggs and maggots, there could not be fewer than one third, or perhaps one half of live young, intermixed a-mong the abortions, which thus inevitably perifhed, I began to re-gret the lofs of fo many induftrious fervants thus deftroyed, when juft emerging into exiftence ; and have, therefore, now laid the practice almoft entirely afide.

of honey, which will make the bees eager of work during the day, and fing for joy through the night. Now is the honey feafon, and farewell famine and robbers; for, when there is honey in the flowers, they will not rob for it; and, a fingle hour of a fine day will refrefh them, and put a period to the labour of feeding them, as formerly hinted.

When the flowers begin to open, the bees will vifit them, and carry off their yellow loads from them. When a loaded bee is feen going into a hive, it is a fign that the flowers are beginning to fpring; and, on every fine day during fpring, fummer, and autumn, they continue to carry on the beloved labour, with the utmoft diligence and alacrity.

The firft day in fpring, that I obferve a bee carrying a load, I generally call my family together, to take a glafs, and rejoice with me and my faithful fervants at the return of the falutiferous feafon. The firft day, perhaps, only three or four loaded bees are to be feen; the next day, probably eight or ten; the third, fifteen; and fo on, the numbers ftill gradually increafing, in proportion to the increafe of the flowers in the fields. The bees then grow

numerous

numerous in the hives; and, about the beginning of May, when the furze and broom,
and many other flowers, make the fields look
yellow, a ftrong hive of bees will be all yellow
loaded; and, at fuch a period, in a fine day,
I have counted 100 loaded bees go into one
hive in a few minutes.

When the hives are all equally good, the
bees carry much alike, but in proportion to
their number. In an apiary, where there are
four hives, one will perhaps have twenty entering into it, in five minutes; another fifty, a
third ninety, and the fourth a hundred and
twenty, all within the fame fpace of time. But
in the height of the honey feafon, the bees carry
amazingly faft, running out and in to the hive
with the moft furprifing celerity and expedition. At this period, the number of loaded bees
conftantly flocking into the hive, as well as their
rapidity, defies all power of calculation; for
although they labour with great affiduity and
conftancy before this feafon, yet they do not
appear to work with fuch incredible quicknefs,
as after the honey feafon commences §.

If

§ In fpring, as the bees gradually increafe in numbers, their
entry fhould be gradually widened, left they fhould be im-
peded

If I were intending to purchafe a hive in May, and came to an apiary where there were four hives, to make choice of one, I would defire four men to fit down for ten minutes, one at each hive, and count the number of loaded bees that entered into their refpective hives in that fpace of time ; and according to their report, I would pitch upon the hive that was moft frequented during that interval, provided it had honey, and were not one of the oldeft.

CHAP.

peded in their labours ; but this fhould only be done in proportion to the number of bees in a hive. During March and April, they fhould be very little, as warmnefs is health to bees, and farthers their hatching greatly. A numerous hive fhould, in May, have an entry two inches wide, and half an inch deep , while a hive, that has not perhaps half the number of bees, fhould have its entry only one inch wide and fcarcely half an inch deep. But in the midft of fummer, when the weather is warm, and the bees numerous, the entries of all the hives fhould be widened, as the bees ought to have both fufficient room to go out and in, and as much air as poffible. In fuch hot weather, the entries might even be enlarged to three inches in widenefs, and one inch in height. The method of enlarging or ftraitening the entries of hives is quite fimple. Pieces of wood, all of one fize outwardly, but with holes cut in the under part of them, of the various dimenfions above defcribed, might be made and kept ready at all times, to be exchanged with each other, according as the feafon requires, or the Bee-mafter wifhes to widen or to ftraiten his hives ; but indeed a little plafter lime will ftraiten or widen an entry in fpring and fummer, with very little trouble.

CHAP. XVIII.

HOW TO UNITE OR RE-INFORCE BEE-HIVES.

As the uniting or re-inforcing of bees is often neceſſary to be performed during the fame feafon of the year, that they naturally fend off young fwarms, thefe two fubjects will often fall to be occafionally intermingled in fuch a manner, that the one cannot be particularly defcribed without taking notice of the other. But as each article is of too much importance, not to require a feparate chapter, and of courfe a *precedence* to one of them, I fhall firft defcribe the UNITING or RE-INFORCING of bee-hives, as it is often neceſſary in different feafons of the year, and fhall devote a fubfequent chapter or two to the fubject of SWARMING.

In handling bees at all times, but efpecially when driving them, or managing a fwarm, gentlenefs and boldnefs are equally neceſſary.

Every

Every motion muft be made deliberately, and
without hurry.   The operator may take a glafs
of good ale, and rub fome of it over his face
and hands ; but during the whole operation he
muft be particularly careful not to bruife any
of the bees.

In uniting and re-inforcing bees,* upon the
very

---

* To RE-INFORCE a hive, fignifies to take part of the bees out
of a ftrong hive, and put them into a weak or deficient one, in order to ftrengthen it, and make it a thriving hive. But one thing
to be obferved here, is, that no bees muft ever be taken from a
ftock hive to re-inforce another with, unlefs in fummer, when the
hive is fo full of bees as to lay out, or nearly fo ; for no good hive
ought at any time to be hurt to enrich a weak one.   It is often
a very neceffary and ufeful operation, when a hive has few bees
in fummer, by re-inforcing her from a more numerous hive
that can eafily fpare them, the weak hive will foon become ftrong.
Or fhould a misfortune befal a hive at any feafon of the year, the
bees of the unfortunate hive fhould be put into another hive ; and
in September, all the bees belonging to the hives which are taken,
fhould be put into the ftock hives, whereby they will preferve heat
through the winter, and be able to accelerate their labours in
the fpring.

In all cafes whatfoever, where it is neceffary to remove the
bees out of one hive into another, the new hive muft be placed
in the fame fpot where the old hive ftood, to prevent the bees from
miftaking it.   But when a hive is re-inforced by an additional
number of bees, if thefe bees are taken from three or four different hives, fituated in as many different places, the re-inforced
hive fhould be removed about a mile diftant from all of them, to
prevent the new inhabitants from returning to their original hives
again ;

very beft plan that I know of, they will fometimes fight a little ; but, although I cannot abfolutely prevent this inconvenience, nor indeed
have I ever met with any author, or feen any
perfon, who could take in hand to do it, yet I
can ufe fuch means, as will probably prevent
any conflict from taking place in one of a dozen
of thefe operations ; and, although a few battles
may occur among fome individual bees, yet
in general very few will be killed on either
fide. I am, therefore, never afraid to unite
them, when I have reafon to believe it will anfwer a good purpofe in other refpects. But,
in all cafes of uniting bees, particular care
fhould be taken firft to try the deficient hive
with a fpecimen of the bees that are intended
to be introduced into it ; and if thefe *ambaffadors* are gracioufly received, the reft of their
brethren may be fafely offered : But, if otherwife, the whole of the bees fhould be kept
back, till thofe of the receiving hive fhall be in

S

better

again. But after ftanding fix weeks, it may be returned back to
its former fituation. The above general directions, I think abfolutely neceffary to be obferved, in driving, re-inforcing, and
fwarming of bees ; and I am perfuaded they will anfwer in moft
cafes, though particular circumftances may occur, wherein the
practical bee-mafter's judgment muft direct him ; as it is impoffible
to anticipate every contingency, in a limited work of this nature.

better humour; for, it is to be remarked, that
the fame bees will often fight at one time, who
will unite in the moft kindly manner at another; on which account the receiving hive
fhould always be previoufly tried, with a fpecimen of their intended new affociates.

To drive all the bees out of a hive, at any
feafon of the year, either to re-inforce another
hive, or to raife an artificial fwarm, the hive
muft be gently turned up, and the top of it
placed in an eek, or in a hole made in the
ground on purpofe, to prevent it from being
overturned. An empty hive of the fame fize
muft then be gently placed over it, mouth to
mouth, and a fheet, or large cloth, wrapped round
the joinings of the hives, to prevent any of the
bees from getting out. The undermoft hive
muft then be rapped with both hands in the
manner a drum is beat; rapping chiefly on thofe
parts of the hive to which the edges of the
combs are fixed, and avoiding the parts oppofite to the fides of the combs, left they fhould
be loofened, and, by falling together, crufh the
bees between them, as well as the young in
the cells. Even the Queen herfelf might be
in danger of fuffering. By not adverting to
this, I have feen the loofe combs and bruifed

bees

bees fall out upon turning up the hive, all of which are a confiderable lofs. The older any hive is, there is the lefs danger of loofening the combs; and the more bees there are in it, the fooner they will run into the new hive; for the concuffion of the hive, by the rapping, alarms them, as an earthquake alarms mankind, and they run to the upper hive in fearch of a more fafe habitation. Thofe that enter firft, finding themfelves fafe, invite their brethren by their founding to follow them, which they quickly do. The fheet may then be removed, and the edge of the upper hive next the right hand lifted up, when, upon a narrow infpection, the Queen fometimes will be obferved to go up along with the reft.

When all the bees are thus removed into the new hive, it may be placed where the old one ftood, which will collect all the bees together, and within ten minutes, they will fall a working as bufily as any natural fwarm.

It is neceffary, before this operation, to remove the hive, eight or ten yards at leaft, from every other hive, to prevent difturbance from other bees. An empty hive fhould alfo be placed where the old hive ftood, to amufe thofe bees belonging to it, that may return loaded from the

fields

fields. This operation may be very eafily performed at any hour of the day; but
the fafeft time is when they are moft bufy at
work, as they are not then fo ready to fting the
operator. In this manner, I have taken off
four artificial fwarms in one forenoon, and
hardly received a fingle fting; for the operation is quite eafily performed, efpecially in the
middle of the day. †

In

---

† Indeed, there is hardly any thing that is requifite to be
done about bees, that I would not take in hand to perform, with
fufficient time and attention.

I could put TWENTY hives, for inftance, into ONE, if neceffary:
I can caufe my bees to rear as many Queens as I pleafe: I can
rob my bees of part of their honey, at any time: I could carry
100 bee hives to LONDON or RUSSIA: I could rear 5,000 bee-
hives in a few years, if defired by any gentleman of property: I could travel through the ftreets of Edinburgh with
three fwarms of bees about me, unhurt: I can take a fwarm out of
any hive at any time: I can take 10,000 bees from ten different hives, and unite them into one hive; and I can re-inforce a weak hive with bees from any number of other hives,
and from being the WORST, make it the BEST hive in the county;
I can unite the bees of forty hives into thirty, twenty, or ten
hives; and next Summer divide thefe ten hives again into forty
fwarms: If I have a weak hive fuffering by robbers, I can
ftrengthen it with more bees, and make them fit to rob any hive
in the neighbourhood: If I have a hive of bees perifhing with
poverty or famine, I can make it the richeft hive in the place, or
within many miles around: I can take a common bee egg, and
caufe

In fummer, a weak hive, that has few inhabitants, may be re-inforced with a number of
bees from a ftrong one, in the following manner : Suppofing there are two apiaries, a mile
diftant from each other ; and that, in one of
them, there are a weak hive and a ftrong one,
fituated within two feet or two yards of each
other ; and no other hive near them : in fuch
a cafe, let the ftrong hive be removed, about
ten o'clock A. M. when the bees are bufy at
work, to twenty or thirty yards diftance, and
let the weak hive be placed where the ftrong
one ftood. All the bees, belonging to the
ftrong hive, that were abroad in the fields, will
thus, on their return, go into the weak hive and
unite peaceably with its inhabitants. Upon
this plan, fcarce one of twenty will fight ; but
if they fhould, which is feldom the cafe when
they are bufy at work, then the ftrong hive
muft be immediately brought back, and placed
in its former fituation ; and the weak hive
turned up and rapped heartily, upon which
the

caufe the bees raife it to be either a Queen or a common bee as I
pleafe : I can make my bees reft upon myfelf or any perfon near
me, without offering us the fmalleft injury ; and I can make
them fall upon us with the fury of as many dragons, fo that we
would be glad to fly with as much precipitation, as a few rioters
would do before a regiment of dragoons.

the bees will return to their own hive again;
and the weak hive may be placed in its former fituation. But when a part of the bees
of the ftrong hive unite peaceably with thofe
of the weak one, the ftrong hive fhould
be carried to the other apiary : for fhould it
be placed too near the fituation where it formerly ftood, too many of its bees might' go into
the weak hive, and thus the one be impover-
ifhed by enriching the other. Another method, to re-inforce a hive with bees, is to bring
it into a clean room, where there is only one
window ; then turn it up, and rap upon it, till
fome hundreds of the bees fly to the light.
They will run up and down the glafs in a bewildered manner, wondering, (we may fuppofe,) how the air has become fo thick, that
they cannot pafs through it. Let them remain
in this fituation for about twenty minutes,
which will cool their courage for fighting.
Then let three or four fcore of thofe bees, that
are wifhed to be united to them, be introduced clofe to them. Thefe will appear as much
bewildered as the former, by the glafs preventing their egrefs, and will readily unite with
them, without killing a fingle bee. Upon finding them thus agree, let them all be brought

to

to the window ; and a fhort time after, let the hive be placed near them, and they will all run into it chearfully : after which the hive, thus re-inforced, may be placed in its former fitua- tion, provided it be about a mile diftant from the place where the old hive formerly ftood. Up- on this plan, even all the combs may be taken out of a hive one by one, during which time, the bees will fly to the window, and a few of, the bees of the receiving hive being made to join them, upon their uniting kindly, the re-. ceiving hive may be placed as above directed.

I have often re-inforced weak hives in fpring, which have done very well, though, at other times, they turned out very indifferently. I therefore feldom attempt to do it now, till the ftrong hives are full of bees, and feem to be near fwarming : on which occafions they can afford 2000 common bees to ftrengthen a weak hive, with very little injury to their own.

Again, in fummer, a weak hive may be re- inforced by changing its fituation with that of a ftrong one, upon a fine day, when the bees are bufily employed at work. I have often practifed this bufinefs with much fuccefs and fatisfaction. But, if they fhould not unite in a friendly manner, let both be turned up, the

ftrange

ftrange bees rapped out, and each hive reftored to its former fituation.

C H A P. XIX.

OF HABITATIONS PROPER FOR BEES TO LIVE AND WORK IN.

HIVES, or the habitations in which bees live, breed and work, have been made of different materials, and in different forms, according to the fancy of people of different ages and countries. MELISSUS, king of Crete, is faid to have been the firft who invented and taught the ufe of bee-hives. Not only ftraw, which experience now proves to be rather preferable to every thing elfe, but wood, horn, glafs, &c. have been ufed for the conftruction of hives. Single box hives, however, when properly made, anfwer very well, and, when painted, laft long. They have feveral advantages above ftraw hives : They are quite cleanly, and always ftand upright; they [are proof againft mice; and are cheaper in the end than ftraw hives; for one

· box

box hive will laft as long as three of them. I
have known many bee-mafters, who never ufed any other kind of hives, and whofe bees
throve very well. I believe, however, they are
rather colder in winter, but a proper covering
will prevent all danger from that quarter. But
ftraw hives are eafieft obtained at firft, and
have been ufed and recommended by the moft
of bee-mafters.

As to the fize, a hive that will hold about 2¼
pecks, Linlithgow meafure, will hold a pretty
large fwarm; but there is no certain rule to
judge what hive will be exactly filled by a
fwarm. Much depends upon the fucceeding
feafon. If the fwarm be early and large, it
will require a large hive; but if otherwife, the
hive fhould be proportionably lefs. If a fwarm
be put into one of the fize above mentioned,
and the bees fill it foon, and appear to want
more room, it can eafily be enlarged, by putting an eek below it: but if it be heavy enough
for a ftock hive, it will do, although it fhould
not be quite full of combs.

A ftraw hive, when made, fhould have a
piece of wood, fixed in the undermoft roll, four
inches long, with a notch cut out of it, three
inches long, and one high, for an entry to the

T

bees

bees. The ftraw of rye or wheat is beft for making hives: The heads of the ftraw fhould be cut off; The rolls fhould be drawn very tight, and wrought together with fmall willows or brambles, fplit and properly dreft, with the pith taken out of them. The hives fhould be made as fmooth as poffible, without leaving any projecting ftraws; which, when not cut or finged away, (as fhould always be done when the hives are rough,) would occafion much unneceffary trouble to the bees, when put into them, to gnaw them off. When the hives are made, and, if neceffary, gently finged with ftraw, four fmall fticks fhould be fixed acrofs the infide of them, at proper diftances, in order not only to keep the hive firm, but alfo to prevent the combs from falling down, (which they would otherwife do by their own weight;) or from being fhifted out of their places, when the hives are rapped upon, or difturbed accidentally.

Some ingenious gentlemen have made their hives to confift of different apartments, though inhabited only by one fwarm. This kind of hives are called COLONIES; but I do not much approve of them; as the partitions prevent that accumulation of heat, which is neceffary

for

for the health of the whole family; and as some of the rooms muſt be colder than others, the bees, eſpecially in winter, will all draw to one place; leaving the other apartments empty, and expoſed to ſuch a degree of cold, as will probably make the honey candy and become uſeleſs. Beſides this method is unnatural, for the bees always lodge in one apārtment, when left to their own liberty, provided it be large e- nough to hold them: and as they lay their eggs in the middle part of their combs and hives firſt, and afterwards gradually enlarge the brood around the centre of the hive, they not only get them more eaſily defended from all danger, but alſo ſooner hatched, by the ſu- perior degree of heat.

Colonies have never yet been, and I am per- ſuaded never will be extended to general uſe, although it is nearly two centuries ſince they were invented by JOHN GEDDY, Eſq. I will not deny, however, that bees may thrive pret- ty well upon this plan; which muſt be allow- ed to have one advantage, as, when properly conſtructed, theſe hives afford an opportunity to the inquiſitive philoſopher of ſeeing the bees carry on their labours. Colony hives are made in various forms, according to the taſte of

T 2   different

different gentlemen. Some confift of three boxes, placed one above another ;' others of an equal number placed collaterally ; and a third kind are made with one box in the front, another behind that, and the third behind the fecond. All thefe different kinds have fquare holes in the fides or tops of the boxes, to allow the bees liberty to go from one box to another, as they may find neceffary; and there are fmall panes of glafs fixed in them, in order to obferve the operations of the bees ; with wooden fhutters to cover the glafs, when it is not intended to infpect the hive.

I have feen, in thofe favourable years when the bees had fwarmed very liberally, that the proprietors have been greatly diftreffed for want of hives, to receive their fecond and fubfequent fwarms. But an experienced beemafter will never be at a lofs in fuch circumftances. If all his empty hives are filled, and if he intends to take honey in Autumn, he will find many other articles in which they will chearfully build and work; fuch as any large jar, half barrel, tub, pot, or box of any kind, that is large enough. For the bees are not delicate in their choice of a habitation; witnefs the well known inftance of SAMSON's dead lion.

lon. They will work in any place during Summer; for although the manufacture of honey and honey combs is fo natural to them, that they can work at no other employment, yet the *fhop* in which they make them, is a matter of indifference to them, provided it is only large enough, and capable of excluding cold, rain and robbers. Even darknefs itfelf is no difparagement, but rather renders their habitation more agreeable to them.

C H A P. XIX.

OF THE NATURAL SWARMING OF BEES.

As it would evidence a confiderable degree of folly to defert an old beaten path, for a new road, unlefs the latter were both nearer and better, fo I would by no means recommend artificial fwarming, if natural fwarms can be obtained. But even, in the latter cafe, many ufeful directions may be given, and fhall be laid down in as plain a manner as poffible.

We

We fhall likewife fhow, how it is fometimes e-
qually neceffary and advantageous to make artificial fwarms, along with the manner of doing it to the beft advantage, when it is neceffary.

As the time when a hive will throw a
fwarm is quite uncertain, efpecially to young
beginners in the bee-hufbandry, a conftant attendance is neceffary in fwarming time, from
eight o'clock in the morning till about three
or four in the afternoon. But this may be
done with little trouble or expence. A boy,
or a girl, or any old perfon, may be employed
to watch the bees during thefe hours ; and this
needs only to be done in fine days, as the bees
feldom fend out a colony in cold, damp, or
chilly weather.

Some hives will ly out long before they fwarm,
though they will fwarm at laft; others, although
they lie out equally long, will not fwarm at
all ; a third clafs will fwarm without the fmalleft previous appearance ; and a fourth will
make a buftle about their doors, for three or
four days before they fwarm : And, therefore,
from fuch a variety of chances, it is fcarce poffible to determine the precife time of fwarming; although we may reafonably conjecture,
from

from the following fymptoms, that this wifhed for period is approaching.

When the number of bees in a hive increafes faft, about the end of May and beginning of June, and drones appear among them; if a fhort time before this, water of an infipid tafte appeared on the ftool, about or within the entry; if this water, which is called *fweat*, and is occafioned by the increafed heat of the hive, be dried up, by the ftill greater increafe of that heat, from the bees becoming more and more numerous; if the bees, about 11 o'clock, A. M. fly about in a reeling manner, making a noife and motion about the front of the hive; all thefe are figns to put the Bee-mafter on his guard, and to prepare him for the joyful event that is faft approaching, of a young colony within a day or two, or even, perhaps, within an hour or two. But if the bees, after all this, run haftily up and down the outfide of the hive, and at laft gather together in a clufter upon the ftool, he may call his friends together, to behold his increafing ftore, as he may depend that they will fwarm immediately: * and nothing can furely be more delightful

ful

* It is indeed furprizing, to fee the young colony leaving their mother

to the bee-master, than to behold the young emigrants flying in the air and darkening the sky with a thousand varying lines.

Mean-time, while he is satisfying his curiosity as to the manner of their swarming, he should observe, whether they are beginning to settle upon any place, in, or near his own apiary,

hive, and deserting it seemingly in the utmost hurry and precipitation, in so much that they can hardly clear the way for each other. A stranger to the nature of these wonderful insects would be apt to conclude, that there was some formidable enemy within, who was murdering them by wholesale, and from whom they were flying for their lives; or else that they were leaving a disagreeable habitation, where there was nothing but war and poverty; and emigrating to some happier situation, where they would enjoy peace and plenty. But the reverse of all this is the truth; for they are going away of their own accord, chearfully parting with their dearest friends, and leaving a warm habitation, and well-stored granary, to seek their fortunes in a new situation, where they will have every thing to provide for themselves, and all the varieties and inconstancy of weather and climate to struggle against.

An old custom still prevails with many, when a swarm of bees are rising, to make a tinkling noise upon a pan, or kettle, as they think that the noise makes them settle the sooner, and prevents them from flying away. But I am of opinion, that when the swarm comes naturally off, it is proper that they should hear and understand each other, which a noise of this kind will prevent. On all such occasions therefore, I use none. But, when the bees attempt to fly off, all kinds of noise should then be used, to frighten and prevent them from hearing each other, and thus incline them to settle at home.

ry, or attempting to fly away, which they they will fometimes do. If the former, he fhould keep at a diftance till they fettle, as going near them might not only prevent them from fettling, but might alfo occafion the death of fome of them, by trampling upon them.

As foon as they alight on any thing, that can eafily be brought to the ground, fuch as the fmall branch of a tree, or a berry bufh, or the like, let a fheet be fpread on the ground near the fwarm, and two fticks placed upon it, a foot afunder. Then place the fwarm upon the fheet, between the fticks, and gently cover it with a hive †, refting the edges of the hive upon the fticks, to prevent it from crufhing any of the bees ; who will thus have free air, and accefs to and from the hive, which muft be covered with a cloth, to prevent the rays of the fun from fcorching the bees, and provoking them to rife and feek out a more comfortable habitation. If their new lodging pleafes them, they will take

U   immediate

---

† Some advife to rub the hive, before it be placed over the fwarm, with a little honey, or fugar and ale mixed, in order to allure the bees. This can do no harm, but I feldom adopt the practice, as I have feen little or no benefit from it ; the Queen getting into the hive is the only allurement to excite the bees to go into it, and alfo to keep them there, when they are gone fafely in.

immediate poffeffion, and fall to work with alacrity. Sometimes, after continuing two or three
hours in it, and beginning to work, they will
rife and fettle on fome other place, or go back
to their mother hive again; and fometimes they
will fly off altogether, in fearch perhaps of a
habitation previoufly fixed on. They muft
therefore be carefully watched till the heat of
the day be over, after which, it may be prefumed, they will not rife again.

As foon as the young colony are fairly lodged
in their new habitation, let the hive be placed
on a ftool, and carried with all due caution to
the place where it is intended to ftand ‡; for
the fooner the hive is ftationed, the fooner the
bees will be acquainted with its fituation. A
few ftragglers, indeed, may fly about the place
where the fheet was firft laid down; but they
will foon either find out the fwarm, or return
to their mother hive, either of which will be no
lofs. When the hive is placed in its proper
ftation

‡ At all feafons, as foon as a fwarm is fairly fettled, both the
fize of the fwarm and the feafon of the year fhould be taken into
confideration. If the fwarm be pretty numerous, if the mother
hive can bear the want of it, and if the feafon be not too far advanced, let it be put into a hive by itfelf. But directions will
afterwards be given, how to act if any of the contrary circumftances occur.

ftation, the cloth fhould be allowed to remain upon it, to keep off the rays of the fun §, till night, when the fkirts may be plaftered over with lime mixed with hair, and thus fixed to the ftool, and the top covered with turf, as formerly directed, page 97.

Sometimes, though feldom, a fwarm will fly off, notwithftanding every method that can be ufed to prevent it. This happens only in very fine calm weather, when the bees have

U 2   had

§ Sometimes, in very hot weather, young fwarms have fuffered greatly, by the intenfe heat melting the wax, and making their combs fall down on the ftool, in confequence of which the honey runs out, the bees are befmeared, the young ones bruifed, and the hive almoft totally ruined. Many hives fuffered in this manner, by the great heat laft fummer, (1794;) but fuch misfortunes only happen in the beft years for honey; and, indeed, it is to be regretted, that we have fo feldom reafon to complain of too much heat.

In fuch favourable years, the beft method to prevent fuch confequences, is to keep the young fwarms, (for the ftock hives are in no danger,) well fcreened from the fcorching rays of the fun, by covering them over on the fouth fide, or placing fcreens before the hives in fuch a manner as to keep off the heat, at the fame time, that they do not obftruct the bees from going out and in to their work. One of the large boards or ftools, which the hives ufually ftand on, being placed on edge upon the ftool before the entry to the hive; but in fuch a pofition that the bees may have free accefs and egrefs, will anfwer this purpofe; and can eafily be removed, as foon as the exceffive heat is over.

had liberty some days before swarming, to
roam about in search of a commodious habitation; which, if once they find, it is difficult,
and often impossible, to prevent them from e-
migrating to it. When the weather is very
favourable, the bees often, before swarming,
send out scouts in search of a proper habitation; and when they discover a hive whose
bees are dead, or any empty place about the
roof of a gentleman's house, or a church, cas-
tle, or trunk of a tree; more especially, if bees
have wrought combs in it the summer before,
but have died out of it in winter, they will
send out a squadron of bees, three or four days
before they swarm, to clean out the place, and
render it fit for the reception of the young colony, the first favourable opportunity. At
such places, I have often seen a considerable
number of bees, busily employed in clearing
away the dead bees, broken crumbs of wax,
and all other rubbish; and sometimes I have observed bees from different hives, laying an equal
claim to the newly discovered habitation, and,
as mankind too often do in similar cases, fighting and killing each other for the uninhabited
territory; for, two swarms have been seen flying

ing to fuch a place in one day, in which cafe
a bloody battle between them often becomes
inevitable.

There have been many inftances of a fwarm
of bees flying in a direct line to a dead hive,
when ·it happened to be within their reach in
a neighbouring-apiary. Such hives are often
left ftanding by the owner, either from his
not knowing that the bees are dead, or from
his ignorance of the confequences. They are
alfo frequently left by roguifh bee-mafters, on
purpofe to entice their neighbours fwarms;
which is as villainous as ftealing a fwarm, if
not more fo. Mr Maxwell fays, there is a law
againft fuffering a dead hive to ftand in an
apiary. If there is, it is a very juft one, but
if not, an act of parliament fhould be paffed
againft fuch a pernicious practice. Such
caufes have been feveral times tried in courts
of juftice, and fome judges have punifhed the
trefpafs, which was certainly juft. But I lately heard of a caufe of this nature, which was
tried before a judge, who affoilzied the aggref-
for, upon this principle, that every man has
a right to keep what he pleafes in his own garden. By this decifion the judge evidenced his
ignorance ; for, if fuch a precedent were

once

once eftablifhed as law, no perfon, who has a covetous bee-mafter in his neighbourhood, would be fure to lofe fome fwarms of his bees ; for, a dead hive, left ftanding in an apiary during fummer, feldom fails to receive a fwarm before Lammas.

Many have been not a little difficulted how to determine, whether the old hive that the fwarm went into, had living bees in it or not, before that event took place. One eafy method of deciding this point, is, by infpecting it, to fee if there are live young in it ; and another is, by the diftance from which the fwarm has come ; for, I know for certain, that a fwarm will not fly a mile to a living hive; whereas, they will fly four miles to take poffeffion of an old one with combs in it, whofe inhabitants are dead. I have, indeed, feen a fwarm go into a living hive, that ftood in the fame apiary ; but this was rather accidental than otherwife. The Queen returning home in confufion, perhaps from a fruitlefs expedition, might miftake another hive for her own. In fuch cafes, a great battle frequently enfues, in which many are flain, and often the Queen among them. Sometimes I have feen them agree very well, and make a good colony, when the hive was

properly

properly raifed with a very large eek. At o-
ther times, I have feen a fwarm, after joining
another hive, being well received, and remaining in it very peaceably, come off, notwithftanding, the very next day.

When a fwarm emigrates, with a view to fettle in fome habitation, which their fpies had
previoufly difcovered, they fly to the place in a
direct line. The bee-mafter fhould, therefore,
run or ride along with them, as far as he can ;
for on fuch occafions they fometimes fly fo flow,
as a perfon who is fwift of foot may accompany
them. But if he fhould be prevented from following them in a direct line, by any interruptions
from woods, waters, or inclofures, let him, upon
recovering the line, proceed ftraight forward,
without turning to the right or left, and the
chance is ten to one that he will difcover them,
efpecially if they happen to alight or reft upon
any dike hedge, or brufh by the way. But
fhould this not happen, upon proceeding ftill
forward, the line will probably lead him to
fome garden where there is an apiary ; the
owner of which fhould be told the cafe ; and
if he is an honeft man, he will doubtlefs allow
his hives to be fearched, in the prefence of wit-
neffes, to fee if the fwarm have taken up their
abode

abode in any of his dead hives. This will eafily be difcovered by examining the entries of his hives, and if there are any fmall crumbs of wax lying like as much faw duft, on the ftool before them, it may be prefumed, that the bees of the new fwarm have cleaned it off the combs; and, therefore, a farther fearch fhould be demanded; and upon turning up the hive, and fearching with a fmall ftick for young bees in the cells, as directed, (p. 129) the matter can foon be decided, whether the hive was inhabited by living bees, previous to the fwarm entering it, or not. If fealed up maggots, or young bees appear in the cells, the owner of the fwarm can have no claim; but if none of thefe appear, he has a right to the hive, which, if the proprietor of the apiary fhould refufe to deliver, he ought to be inftantly fummoned before a Magiftrate, while the hive is ftill totally deficient of young bees; when the cafe being plainly ftated, and *this decifive proof* adduced, the young fwarm will doubtlefs be ordered to be reftored, and the greedy proprietor of the dead hive in all probability fined for his covetoufnefs.

But if the fwarm fhould not have alighted at the firft apiary in the direct line, the owner fhould ftill proceed ftraight forward, and he
                                                will

will in all probability arrive at another apiary,
where the fame inquiries and mode of inveftigation fhould be repeated : Or if any hollow
tree,, church, gentleman's manfion-houfe, old
ruin, or any other building, fhould happen to
lie in the direct line, they fhould be infpected
attentively, and proper inquiries made at the
people in the neighbourhood, if they obferved
a fwarm of bees flying or fettling on any of
them. By thefe means perfevered in, a difco-
very will certainly be made ; and if the fwarm
has fettled in any fuch place, the following directions will fhow the method of taking them
out in this and other cafes of a like nature. If
a fwarm fettle in a hollow tree, or any cavity of a building, it will be impoffible to get it
out by any other means, than taking them out
by handfuls. Some indeed, alledge, that rapping will force them out ; but not one fwarm
of twenty will yield to that method, unlefs the
Queen can be laid hold of, and brought out.
The owner fhould, therefore, make as much
room as poffible, to get his hand introduced, fo
as to pull them out by handfuls, and put them
into an empty hive ; and as foon as he is fo fortunate as to get hold of the Queen, he fhould
put her into the hive, where fhe will prevent

X the

the bees from ftraying; and thofe that were ftill remaining in the building or hollow tree, will quickly come to the hive, and join the reft. In fuch cafes, I have fearched whole hours for the Queen, who generally hides herfelf with fo much art, that it is extremely difficult to lay hold of her, although in fuch fearches I feldom failed to catch her at laft. But when the Queen cannot, by any means, be got, and when all or the greateft part of the fwarm is recovered, let the hole be clofe fhut up, and a weak hive brought, and re-inforced with the common bees, (as directed page 142) which is the beft ufe that can be made of them in fuch cafes.

Before bees fwarm the fecond or third time, they do not ly out in clufters about the hive or upon the ftool; but as foon as they are ready, they come off in a body, even in weather that is by no means favourable. The figns, when thefe after fwarms will come off, are more cer-tain than thofe that precede the firft fwarm-ing; for, if the weather be good, one may al-moft prognofticate the very hour. By liften-ing at night to the found of a hive, about eight, ten, or twelve days, after the firft fwarm is gone off, that peculiar found, commonly called *toll-ing*, will be eafily diftinguifhed. This found

feems

feems to be the royal proclamation iffued by the young princefs, to warn, or rather to invite her fellow emigrants to prepare for their intended journey. It founds, fays one, as if the words *peep! peep! peep!* were rapidly pronounced fifteen or twenty times in half a minute. She then ftops, and begins again repeatedly, like a chicken peeping for its mother, when it has loft her. When there are feveral young Queens in the hive, there will be fo many diftinct voices repeating this call. I have fometimes heard thefe princeffes calling from all corners of the hive ; and, as it were, anfwering each other ; fome calling out *peep, peep,* in a treble voice, and others anfwering in a voice rather more hoarfe, and comparatively like bafs *. When thefe founds are heard

X 2   in

---

* Almoft all authors agree, that thefe peculiar voices proceed from the young Queens *petitioning* (fo to fpeak,) for *leave* to emigrate with a young fwarm. I have fometimes thought, however, that this noife might alfo proceed from fear or rage being excited amongft them. I was led to entertain this opinion, by obferving their different fcreams one day, which made me fufpect that there were more than one Queen in the hive. And as I wifhed to have one or two of them to enable me to caufe fome out-laying hives fwarm, I drove all the bees out of that hive. One Queen went along with them ; but I ftill perceived other two Queens, befides three royal cells fealed up. I ftill heard the ufual quick cry of the Queen ; and, upon attentively obferving their motions;

in the hive, the emigration of a fwarm may be depended upon, within a day or two at moft, if the weather holds tolerably good. The firft night that thefe founds are obfervable, they are low, and not very frequent, nor even the next day; but, on the fecond night, they become louder and more frequent, in fo much that they may fometimes be diftinguifhed at the diftance of fome yards from the hive. Next day, if the weather be favourable, a fwarm may be depended upon. "It is delightful, (fays Mr THORLEY) to hear thofe peculiar and " mufical founds or notes, being an eight or " chord, which is truly harmonious." They are fcarcely ever heard before a firft fwarm goes off; I believe not once in fixty cafes. The reafon, I fuppofe, is, that they have in ge-neral, only one Queen reared to go off with the firft fwarm; and fometimes, when tempt-ed by very fine weather, even the old Queen will go off with the firft colony, before the

young

tions, I faw them going to the royal cells, and tear at them with great fury, fcreaming and roaring feemingly with great indigna-tion :—a phænomenon, which I could only account for, upon the principle of their entertaining a jealoufy left their rivals in the cell fhould fome forward, and ftand in competitition with them

young princefs comes out of the royal cell. *
Whereas, before the fecond or third emigration takes place, they will fometimes have two
or three Queens, and as many royal cells, in
their hive; one of which may be taken to fupply any hive that needs them.

Often have I feen a young Queen take an
airing. For inftance, in Summer 1790, I had
a hive that had no Queen in it, but a pregnant
royal cell, which had been feven days fealed
up; on which account, I expected that a

Queen

---

* The Queens are generally bred in fwarming time, as may
be obferved by turning up a hive at that period, when the royal
cells may be perceived on the edges or fides of the combs, although fometimes they hang from the middle. Thefe cells are
of an oblong circular form, of confiderable thicknefs, and in appearance rather clumfy. One of them will weigh as much as
four or five fcore of common cells. When half made, they are
not unlike the lower part of an acorn, turned upfide down; they
gradually lengthen, and, when finifhed and fealed up, are about
an inch in length, and would refemble the end of one's little
finger, if it wanted the nail. In fwarming time, there will fometimes be from one to fix of thefe royal cells; though commonly
there are not above two or three. They all hang perpendicu-
larly, with their open ends pointing downwards to the ftool.
After the young Queens are hatched, thefe cells are fometimes
removed by the bees, and fometimes allowed to remain; but I never faw an egg laid in an old cell to be a Queen; for the bees
always build a new cell when they want a young Queen.

Queen would foon emerge out of the cell. And, as I was anxious to fee what appearance fhe made the moment of her birth, I turned up the hive every hour, and luckily hit the time that fhe was opening the cell for herfelf, when I faw her come out of it, and creep about pretty well. Two days thereafter, I faw her come to the entry of the hive, and fly off and take an airing. She returned within about ten minutes thereafter, and went back into the hive, where the bees received her with joy. I have alfo feen many other young Queens do the fame on the fecond or third day of their age. Perhaps old ones may do fo too; but I think this happens very feldom, as they are large and heavy, and confequently may be afraid to truft themfelves to their wings. No doubt, the old Queens can fly when they pleafe, although, like many old people, they are not very fond of much travel.

It will fometimes happen, in an apiary where there is a confiderable number of bee-hives, that two fwarms will go together in the time of fwarming, when they chance to come out of their mother hives nearly about the fame time. When one fwarm is nearly fettled on a bufh, hedge, or any other place, and another begins

to

to come off from the mother hive, the mufic of the former invites the latter to join them. In fuch circumftances, therefore, the moft effectual method to prevent the junction of the two fwarms, is to cover the firft fwarm completely with a large fheet, which will prevent the other fwarm from hearing their melody. But if the firft fwarm be got into a hive, or nearly all entered, it fhould be carried into a houfe, and kept there for fome little time, till the fecond fwarm be fairly fettled fomewhere ; after which the hive fhould be brought back to its former fituation. But when both fwarms are fmall, or but of a medium fize, if they unite voluntarily and peaceably together, as they generally do in fuch cafes, their junction will be rather an advantage than a lofs : For it is certain, that 16,000 bees in one hive will collect more honey and wax than the fame number of bees lodged in two different hives could poffibly do*.

CHAP.

---

* This can be eafily accounted for. In every hive there is a certain number of bees appointed to hatch the young, and to defend the hive from robbers, &c. Now, fuppofing that each hive requires 2,000 bees to be daily occupied in thefe employments, then it follows, that 16,000 bees; lodged in two different hives, muft devote 4,000 of their number to thefe objects, and

leave

CHAP. XXI.

,OF THE ARTIFICIAL SWARMING OF BEES.

ALTHOUGH, in moſt caſes, bees are beſt directed by natural inſtinct, and on that account

I

leave only 12,000 at work in both hives, whereas, the ſame number of bees in ONE hive, requiring only 2,000 to be devoted to theſe employments, will allow 14,000 to be conſtantly employed in the fields, and of courſe one ſeventh part more honey and wax may be produced in the courſe of the ſeaſon. There are alſo other advantages ariſing from ſuch a junction of ſmall ſwarms: They require, for inſtance, only one place in the garden; being more in number; they afford more heat to bring forward the young, and they are more able to defend the hive from robbers, &c. &c.

And here it may be both uſeful and entertaining, to take notice of the various weights and numbers of different ſwarms. "It "has been found, (ſays BUTLER,) that a larger number than "40 or 50,000 will not thrive together in one hive. Swarms "often amount to 30,000; a large ſwarm may weigh eight "pounds, and gradually leſs to one pound; conſequently a "very good one weighs five or ſix pounds, a moderate one "four pounds. No ſwarms leſs than this ſhould be kept, but "united with others." If we conſider that about 5000 bees weigh a pound, a ſwarm weighing four pounds, will have near about 20,000 bees, which will compoſe a very good ſwarm. But I am of opinion, that a ſwarm, conſiſting of 15,000 bees, will do very well in a ſingle hive, if the ſeaſon is not too far advanced; and, indeed, the more numerous the ſwarm is, ſo much the better. I myſelf have had above 30,000 bees in one ſwarm.

I am always beft pleafed with natural fwarms, yet it may be obferved of them, as well as of moft other animals, intended for the ufe or benefit of man, that confiderable room is left for human art and ingenuity to affift them. Thus, for inftance, they are provided by human art with much more convenient habitations, than they could either rear or difcover by their own inftinct : For, without our aid, if no ruinous houfe or hollow tree were near, a young fwarm might hang on a bufh, till they were either totally deftroyed by wind, or drowned by rain. Artificial fwarming, therefore, when a natural fwarm (which is always preferable,) cannot be obtained, is fometimes a neceffary and ufeful part of bee hufbandry ; and will, indeed, turn out ultimately to our own advantage, as will appear from what follows.

Before proceeding farther, however, with any directions on this fubject, it is proper to caution the reader, that although artificial fwarming is very profitable, when properly performed by an experienced bee-mafter, yet it always has been, and ever will be, very deftructive to bees, if performed by unfkilful perfons: and, indeed, all new beginners may

Y

be almoft certain of ruining fome hives in their firft attempts. But, by carefully obferving the following directions, the moft inexperienced bee-mafter may foon come to the practical knowledge of the art, and thereby avoid fuch blunders as would prove deftructive to his bees.

CASE I, Sometimes, when two fwarms meet, a dreadful battle enfues, on account of there being two Queens among them. Each party feems determined to defend their own Queen and mother at the rifk of their lives. Their fury generally lafts till one of the Queens is flain, after which a peace commonly takes place, and the two bands unite harmonioufly in one community*.

But

---

* In thefe conflicts, it is aftonifhing to fee what dreadful havock they make in a very fhort time. In my younger years, I have feen above 1000 of thefe brave winged foldiers lying weltering in their gore, within the fpace of ten minutes. The Queen of one or both fwarms is often feized inftantaneoufly, and murdered. On fuch occafions, I have feen above an hundred bees, all wrapt together in a clufter, of the fize of a fmall apple, and fo firmly compacted together around the body of a Queen, that it was with the utmoft difficulty I could feparate them from her. Moft writers are of opinion, that the bees, which thus clufter round a Queen, are her enemies, and that their being fo clofely compacted together about her proceeds from the keen enmity

of

But, if they do not unite in a friendly manner, there is not a moment to be loft. The
hive muft be inftantly turned up, and the bees
driven into four or five different hives. Every
clufter of them muft be fearched for the
Queen, who, when caught, muft be feparated from all the other bees, whether friends or
foes, as, at fuch a time, it is impoffible to diftinguifh the one from the other. And, while
fhe is kept clofe prifoner, the bees may be
frightened from farther fighting; and even
gradually pacified, by rapping on the hives,
and thus driven out of one hive into another.
If this attempt does not fucceed to bring the
bees to a good underftanding with each other,
cold water may be fprinkled on them in the
hives to cool their courage; or they may be
taken into a room, as directed, page 142, and
when, by their being thus toffed and tumbled
about, (all due care being taken, however, not

Y 2   to

___

of each to be firft at her with his dagger. It is, indeed, beyond
a doubt, that Queens are often furrounded in this manner by
their enemies, who frequently kill them very quickly. But I
am of opinion, that they are often likewife encompaffed by their
friends in a fimilar manner, whofe loyal zeal for their fovereign
mother leads them thus to form an impregnable phalanx around
her with their bodies, to protect her perfon from the rage of her
moft inveterate foes.

to hurt them) their spirits are brought low, they may be put into two different hives, and a Queen offered to each. To try their temper, however, a specimen of the bees may be first introduced to the Queen, and if they treat her with mildness, she may then be introduced to the whole swarm. But, if they appear to be still in bad humour, the Queen should be kept back till they become more pacific, which they will quickly do; for as soon as they get leisr e to think, they will miss their Queen, and make all possible enquiry after her, running up and down the hive with the utmost impatience and anxiety, in search of their sovereign mother; and, when they cannot discover her any where, they will conclude that she has perished during the tumult, and most of them will creep out of the hive in despair, and crawl about on the ground till they die; their case being quite desperate, as they have not an egg to raise another Queen from. Some will perhaps attempt to fly home, hoping to find their mother there; and others will try if they can gain admittance into any other hive. This is the critical moment to present a Queen to them. As soon as a few of them discover her, they will surround her with the greatest

pleasure

pleafure, and fing aloud for joy. The reft, hearing the joyful news, will all crowd around her, and be ready to fuffocate her in their extacy. She fhould then be placed on the ftool, as in other cafes; but if, during the conflict, one or both Queens have been killed, the bees may either be reftored to their original hives, or put into any others where they fhall be moft favourably received.

In this laft fpring, (1795,) having two hives, that had but few bees in each, I put the bees of the one hive into the other; fufpecting, that as they had both bred flowly, there might be a defect in the health of one or both of their Queens; and hoping that, by putting them together, the bees would probably hold a confultation, which of the two Queens was moft healthy, and, after electing her, kill or banifh the other, as they thought proper. The common bees of both hives at once united kindly and feemed happy; but, upon turning up the hive within 20 minutes after, to fee if all was well, I perceived a few bees cluftered together, which, however, did not greatly furprife me, as I thought the conjoined republics had already decided, which Queen fhould remain in the hive, and that thefe bees were leading the

rejected

rejected Queen to exile or execution. But, u-
pon a more close inspection, I obſerved the two
Queens ſtruggling together with the utmoſt
fury, and darting the moſt deadly blows at each
other. Being afraid of loſing both, and thereby
ruining the united hive, by their mutually killing each other, which muſt have been the
caſe, had one of them thruſt her ſting into the
other's body and left it, as ſometimes happens,
though rarely *, among the common bees in
ſuch conflicts, I ſeparated them, and kept them
aſunder, though they ſtill ran with great fury
in ſearch of each other along the table §. I then
took

---

* Inſtances of this do not happen above once, perhaps, in fifty
times; although the fact is certain, that they ſometimes kill
themſelves, by leaving their ſtings in the bodies of their oppon-
ents.

§ The above-mentioned battle, between the two Queen
Bees, reminded me, at the time, of thoſe lines in the old ſong
of Chevy-Chace; where the brave DOUGLAS is repreſented as
ſaying,

   " But truſt me, PIERCY, pity it were,
    " And great offence to kill
   " Any of theſe, our harmleſs men,
    " For they have done no ill.

   " Let you and I, the battle try,
    " And ſet our men aſide,"
   " Then c—ſt be he, (quoth Earl PIERCY,)
    " By whom it is denied."

took the one that appeared to be the boldeſt, and put her again into the hive, where ſhe was kindly received by the bees, and put the other Queen into another hive, to be dealt with, as the bees might incline, as I had no other uſe for her at that ſeaſon.

Let not my readers, from this account, ſuppoſe, that the common bees are a race of cowards, who will ſtand regardleſs and indifferent, while their ſovereigns or mothers are in danger. On the contrary, they are a ſet of brave and *patriotic* warriors, who will riſk their lives in defence of their hive, their property, or their ſovereign mother. But, when a *duel* takes place between two Queen bees, they commonly, nay almoſt always, diſpatch one of the Queens themſelves.

CASE II. If the rays of the ſun have been intercepted by a cloud, or a ſhower of rain has occurred in the time of ſwarming, the ſmallneſs of the ſwarm may be aſcribed to theſe circumſtances having prevented the half of the young colony from leaving the mother hive. In this caſe, let the ſwarm be placed where the original hive ſtood, for about a quarter of an hour, in which time, the bees that are returning from the fields, will ſoon make the

ſwarm

fwarm large enough, and then the fwarm fhould be removed to about a mile diftance, to prevent the bees from going back to the old ftock again.*

CASE III. When a perfon has a fmall fwarm, whether it be a firft, fecond or third one, and at the fame time a lying-out hive, that has been long in fwarming, he fhould drive all the bees out of the lying-out hive, into an empty one, (fee the method, page 138) and fet down the bees in the fame fpot where they ftood formerly, which will make a fine large artificial fwarm, as fuch a hive would have abundance of bees ; after which, let the fmall fwarm be put into the old hive, where they will hatch out all the young, and make a good hive ; and let the old hive be placed on the fame fpot where the fmall fwarm ftood.

CASE

* When bees come naturally off in a fwarm, they take a view of the place where they fettle, and never think of going back to their mother hive ; but, when they are feparated from their mother hive by driving, or when the hive is fhifted from where it formerly ftood, they are infenfible of the change of their fituation, and always fly back to their former ftation; for, which reafon, the bee-mafter fhould always remove every artificial fwarm, or re-inforced hive, to fome confiderable diftance, otherwife a number of the bees will go back again.

CASE IV. If there are two fmall fwarms, but no hives, that have bees fufficient either to exchange with, or re-inforce them, let them be united; for, in fuch cafes, two fwarms, conjoined into one, will profper better, and turn out more profitable, than three fmall ones kept feparate. See page 167.

CASE V. Suppofe one drive all the bees out of a hive, and thereby make an artificial fwarm, if the old hive has a royal cell in it, by introducing about 5000 common bees into it, they will hatch out the young Queen, with all the eggs and nymphs (or young bees) in the cells, and render it a flourifhing hive. The method of introducing the common bees, is as follows: Let a ftrong lying-out hive be removed from its ufual fituation, about 10 A. M. and place the hive that has no bees on the fpot where it ftood. The bees, on their return from the fields, will enter it, and will no doubt be furprized at the fudden revolution, having left their hive full of their brethren, not one of whom is now to be feen; but, finding plenty of honey, and abundance of eggs, they will make the beft of their misfortune, and fpeedily replenifh the hive, by rearing up the young bees, and working with as much alacrity, if not more, than when they

Z were

were in their original hive. It will be neceffary, however, in this operation, to remove the
original hive to another apiary, (See p. 176.)

CASE VI. When one has a hive that has long
lien out, and ftill fhows no appearance of fwarming, if a fwarm is wifhed for, all the bees may
be driven out, as directed, page 138. A fwarm
may thus be obtained, which, if the weather
anfwers, will not fail to fucceed. The old hive
may be placed below fome other hive, the bees
whereof will hatch out the young bees, and in
autumn the honey may be taken out of it, and
all the bees put into the upper hive.

CASE VII. I have often formerly taken all the
bees out of a hive to make an artificial fwarm,
and put into it a confiderable number of common bees, in order to hatch out the young
brood in the combs, build a royal cell, and rear
a Queen for themfelves. This practice I found
in general anfwered very well, as the bees hardly ever failed to rear a Queen. The only objection againft it arifes from this confideration,
that from the time the old Queen is taken a-
way, till the young one is fit to lay eggs, a period of twenty five days elapfes, during which
time there is not a fingle egg laid in the hive.
And when it is farther confidered, that there
                                        muft

muft be an additional lofs of other 18 days, before the eggs can be bees for any ufe, it is evident, that the beft part of the honey feafon will be over, and confequently that by autumn, the hive will be greatly deficient in bees. For thefe reafons I have now almoft entirely given up the practice, though I have fometimes had hives that profpered very well under it. And, indeed, if I intended to kill a hive of bees in autumn, I would rather prefer the taking away their Queen from them about the end of July, and leaving a great number of common bees in the hive, which, as they would have few bees to nurfe up, would collect a greater quantity of honey in that period, than if they had a Queen in the hive daily laying eggs for them, which would employ a good number of the bees, both to hatch and nurfe up the young, and the re- by, the fewer would be employed in collecting honey.

CASE VIII. If a fwarm fhould come off, which the mother hive cannot afford to want without great injury, it ought to be returned again into the old hive, in this manner : Take the Queen from the new fwarm and confine her in a box; and then turn up the hive containing the new fwarm, and place it before the entry of the old

ftock

ftock which the bees came from, in fuch a manner that the bees in it may run from it into the entry of the old hive again; which they will foon cheerfully do, efpecially as their Queen was taken from them. This operation is fo eafy that it may almoft be performed by a child.

CASE IX. When the fummer is far advanced, and it may be rather late for fwarming, an eek, placed below a ftrong hive, will give the bees more room to work, and may prevent a late fwarm from coming off, which, in general, turns out more lofs than advantage to the Bee-mafter.

C H A P. XXII.

OF THE KILLING OF DRONES.

IT is a good fign that a hive is thriving, and a certain proof that there is a Queen in it, when the working bees kill their drones early: for in thofe hives that have loft their Queen, the bees become fo carelefs both about their honey

and

and their hive, that they permit the drones to live till November or December. And perhaps there is no fmall wifdom in this, for the bees, knowing that they cannot breed any more, are probably fenfible, that they will gain more by the additional heat of the drones preferving them from the feverity of the winter, than they will lofe by the expence of maintaining them; and confequently lengthen out their own lives, as well as thofe of the drones.

This leads me to think, that the drones are not fo fhort-lived as is generally believed. If the working bees did not kill them in the end of fummer and beginning of harveft, but left them to die of old age, they might perhaps live in a good warm hive till fpring. The bees feldom begin to kill the drones, till the honey feafon be nearly over. When, therefore, the maffacre of the drones begins, one may know that, in general, the honey is becoming rather fcarce in their neighbourhood; although it is not an infallible fign; for the bees of fome hives kill their drones fooner than thofe of others, ftanding in the fame apiary. In hives fituated near early paftures, when the flowers are moftly gone, the bees will kill their drones in the end of July. In later fituations, they are permited to
live

live till Auguft. During this laft autumn, (1794,) I faw many excellent thriving hives, fituated among good heath, whofe drones were not extirpated till about the end of September.

As the working bees, when the flowers become fcarce, kill the drones, and thus fhow us plainly, that they are now become ufelefs in the hive ; fo I agree with almoft every writer on this fubject, that it is proper to affift the bees in extirpating them. The manner in which the working bees kill the drones is this. They not only fting them, but pull and bite them with their teeth. It is incredible what havock they will make of them in a fingle day, as I have often been convinced, by obferving great numbers of them lying dead before the door of the hive ‡. They alfo fometimes

‡ When the bees once fall a-killing the drones, it is amazing to fee how intent they are on the bufinefs.—They not only difpatch the old ones, but they alfo tear out and deftroy the young drone-maggots in the cells,—efpecially in bad weather. I have indeed feen them, even before fwarming time, when it had been wet weather for five or fix days, become fo difconfolate, fo difcouraged, and even defperate, (thinking, perhaps, that the weather would never mend,) that they threw out, before the entry of their hive, fome fcores of white young drones ; but, on the return of fair weather,—inftead of tearing out and killing the remainder of this unfortunate race, the Queen immediately

times kill them in a more tedious and linger-
ing, but no lefs effectual way, by banifhing
them from their granaries of honey ; upon
which the drones retreat in great numbers to
the ftool and the under edges of the hive ; and
fometimes, though rarely, I have even feen
them come to the outfide of the hive, in fmall
clufters. When thus exiled, they foon become
very dull and lifelefs, and at laft die for want of
food.   Upon lifting up a hive from the ftool,
I have obferved numbers of them fitting clofe
upon it, with hardly three or four common
bees among them, and on fuch occafions I
have trode to death forty, or more of them, at
once, with my foot.   But, without lifting the
hive,

diately laid frefh eggs, in the drone cells, and the common bees
again carefully reared them up to maturity.

   Whenever, therefore, the young drones are torn out of their
cells before fwarming time, in bad weather, the bees ought immediately to be fed, which will prevent them from defpairing,
and fave the lives of the young drones.

   It is alfo neceffary to mention, that if the weather be bad for
two or three days, after a new fwarm is introduced into an empty
hive, the bees fhould be fed and encouraged by a little honey ;
as, in fuch cafes, I have frequently feen them, when long confined, not only foon difcouraged, but fome of them die ; whereas, by being carefully fed, they are not only kept in good
fpirits, but will, with greater chearfulnefs, embrace the firft favourable moment for refuming their labours.

hive, any perfon may eafily affift the working
bees to kill the drones, (as foon as the bees fhow
us the example), by fitting down at the fide
of the hive the firft good day thereafter, about
eleven o'clock, and crufhing them one by one,
as they come out of the hive, by prefling them
to the ftool with his fore finger. In this manner, an hundred drones may be killed in a very
fhort time. I generally kill the moft of the
drones in my hives when I have leifure ; although there is no abfolute neceffity for doing it, as the working bees will perform the
tafk themfelves in due time. But it certainly
occafions a confiderable faving of honey, and
I am inclined to think, that no harm can a-
rife from it, efpecially in thofe hives whofe
honey is to be taken in Autumn. However,
when there are very few drones in a hive I kill
none of them ; but when they are very numerous, I often kill fome hundreds ; at leaft two
thirds of them, and leave the working bees to
kill the reft at their leifure.

CHAP.

C H A P. XXIII.

ADVANTAGES OF CHANGING THE SITUATION OF BEE-HIVES
TO BETTER PASTURE.

ABOUT Lammas, thofe who live in fituations where the vegetation is early over, efpecially if poffeffed of a large number of hives,
ought to remove their bees to the neighbourhood of heath grounds, if they fhould even
be fix or eight miles diftant, and allow them
to continue in that fituation till the heath gives
over bloffoming. This meafure 1 would earneftly recommend, as the bees, after having
had all the advantage of their early fituations,
will work as late in the feafon, as thofe in the
lateft fituations. I have often feen a hive, by
being placed nigh heath, become ten, twelve,
or fifteen pounds heavier, in the month of Auguft; ‡ whereas, if it had remained in its ori-

A a   ginal

‡ I can affure my readers, that, in the middle of September
1792, I have feen bees in fuch fituations, filling their hives
with combs and honey, as plentifully and as expeditioufly,.

as

ginal early fituation, it would probably have become every day lighter after Lammas. The only rifk in this cafe is, that if the weather turn out bad in Auguft, the bee-mafter will lofe all his trouble; but contingencies of this kind happen in every other bufinefs in which mankind engage, which neverthelefs do not deter us from adventuring.

When bees are placed in a new fituation, they fhould not be permitted to come out of their hives, for the firft time, in cold weather; for, finding themfelves in a ftrange place, they will fly about and take a view of the neighbourhood; and fome of them alighting, and refting on the cold ground, the cold benumbs them, and they perifh, unlefs fpeedily recovered by the heat of the fun. When I remove a hive to a new ftation, I keep them clofe prifoners till the firft fine day, when, about 10 o'-clock A. M.—the time they are moft impatient

to

as if it had been the middle of June. In the beginning of September, that year, I purchafed for a gentleman in Northumberland, a confiderable number of hives, that were only about half full of combs when placed in his apiary; but the heath in his grounds being extremely rich and in full bloffom, the bees were fo expeditious in their labours, that they filled the hives completely with both combs and honey, within a week thereafter.

to get out, I place a feeding comb before their
entry, which I at the same time open, and the
bees come out in great numbers, and fly about
with great alacrity, making their usual chear-
ful music in the air, for two or three minutes,
and taking a view of their new situation. In
the mean time, some of them discover the feeding comb, and entertain themselves with it,
while the flying bees alight at the entry, and
make their usual music for joy; which invites
the straggling bees to return home, so that,
perhaps, scarce a single bee of the whole hive
will have missed its way; whereas, if they are
allowed to go out singly, especially in cold
weather, a considerable number of bees will
be lost, for want of such music in the air, or
at the entry of the hive, to call them home.

In the removal of bees in general, it is better
and safer, to remove a hive to the distance of a
mile or so, than to a nearer situation; for, when
a hive is removed out of an apiary, where there
are a considerable number of hives, to the distance of about a quarter of a mile or so; and es-
cially, if the bees are allowed to come gradually
out of their hives, they will fly to their old place
of abode; but not finding their own hive, they
will fly about in search of it, in a disconsolate

manner

manner, for hours perhaps ; and after being repeatedly difappointed, they will at laft try thofe
hives that ftand neareft the place where their
own hive ftood, to fee if the inhabitants will
admit them, as fo many *deftitute orphans,* into
their community. When they thus come in
a humble fupplicating manner, they are feldom
refufed permiffion to enter, and affociate with
the reft of the hive, as fellow-labourers. Being favourably received, they are ever after
treated, not only as *allies*, but as *brethren* of the
fame family, and live in the greateft harmony
with them ever after.

Similar meafures ought to be adopted in all
cafes of uniting and re-inforcing whatever.
If any perfon fhould take a hive out of his
own apiary, and drive all the bees out of it,
they would fly about in the fame manner, and
at laft enter into thofe hives, that would admit
them kindly. In fuch cafes, however, the firft
ambaffadors, (like thofe of King DAVID to
HANUN, the Ammonite,) may, perhaps, be
miftaken for SPIES, and treated accordingly.
But it will fometimes happen, that the bee-
mafter is in fuch circumftances, that he will be
obliged to remove a hive a quarter of a mile
from other bees. In this cafe, he muft keep
the

the bees prifoners for fome time, as above-mentioned, efpecially if the hives in the original appiaries be fhut or covered over, till the bees of the removed one fly about for an hour or fo. Thus, the lofs will be the lefs, as perhaps fome of the ftraggling bees may find their way back to their own brethren again. But even although an hundred, or two hundred bees fhould fly off in this manner, a ftrong hive will fuffer little by the want of them.

CHAP. XXIV.

OF BEE-BREAD AND WAX,

THE fubftance, commonly called BEE-BREAD, is to be found at the bottom of many of the cells, and is frequently covered over with honey. The bees carry it home in loads upon their legs, or rather their thighs. It is generally of a yellow colour, but often takes its colour from the flowers from which it is collected.

Various

Various conjectures have been made by different authors refpecting its ufe. Some alledge that the bees eat it ; hence the name, *Bee-bread.* Others fuppofe, that, after being taken into their ftomachs, it is converted by fome peculiar action of their internal juices into wax, of which every body knows their combs are made. But an objection to this hypothefis, arifes from the confideration, that the bees, when firft put into an empty hive, carry little or none of this ftuff on their legs for fome time, till a great number of combs are made ; and that after the combs are completed, (which they generally are within two or three weeks after the fwarm have taken poffeffion of the hive,) the bees ftill continue to carry in this ftuff during the whole working feafon. To this, however, it may be replied, that perhaps, as they have no cells to put it into at that time, they carry it home in their bellies, where it probably undergoes a fpeedy change in paffing through their bodies, and may thereby be converted into perfect wax, with which they manufacture their combs.

There is another clafs of authors, who fuppofe that the bee-bread is ufed by the old bees to feed the young ones in the cells, by the

mouth

mouth, as pigeons feed their young ones. To this it may be objected, that the young bees furely cannot make ufe of all the bee-bread, which the old bees are almoft conftantly carrying into the hive when they are at work. Perhaps both thefe laft hypothefes may be true ; as it may not only ferve to feed the young bees, but alfo, by paffing through the bodies of the old ones, may be converted into wax ; with which bees not only build their combs, when a fwarm is newly put into a hive, but alfo feal up both their young in the cells, and their honey in the combs. If this fuppofition be true, then the confumption of bee-bread, through the courfe of the year, but efpecially during the honey and breeding feafons, muft be very great; and therefore we need not be furprized at the quantities imported by the working bees. But, whatever truth may be in either or both of thefe theories, I am certain of one thing, that the bees do not live on beebread alone ; for they will die of hunger, although there be plenty of it in the hive, if there be no honey in it; whereas, when they have abundance of honey, théy will live without bee-bread, at leaft for many weeks. REAU-
MUR

MUR, however, fays, that it is abfolutely neceffary for food to bees.

For my part, I have always obferved the bees
moft bufily employed in carrying in this ftuff
while the young bees are breeding; but when
they want a Queen, and have no eggs to rear
another, they immediately give over carrying
it into the hive, thinking, (as it would feem,)
that as they have no young bees to feed or feal
up in the cells, it would be an idle bufinefs to
bring any more of it home, efpecially as they
do not make much ufe of it themfelves, and
have more already in the hive than they will
ftand in need of, for their own ufe. MR
THORLEY alledges, that the bees carry the wax
home from the fields in fine fmall fcales‡ between the folds of their bodies. He fays, that
" For feveral feafons, after I became a Bee-ma-
" fter, I was very defirous and diligent to find
" out how, or where, they brought home their
" wax, well knowing that grofs matter to be of
" a very contrary nature, and applied to fome
                                  " other

‡ Thefe fcales are well known by bee-mafters, and fomewhat
refemble fmall falt at a diftance, but, upon a nearer infpeftion,
they are more like the fcales of very fmall fifh, being thin, fmall,
round and white. Their fubftance is nothing but pure wax.

" other ufe, but was not able for a confiderable
" time, to enter into the fecret.

" At laft, viewing a hive of bees very bufy
" at labour, I obferved one bee among the reft,
" as fhe fixed upon the alighting place, of an
" unufual appearance ; upon which I feized
" her directly, before fhe had time to enter the
" hive ; where, with a very fenfible pleafure, I
" found what I had (till then) been in vain
" fearching for. Upon the belly of this bee,
" within the plaits, were fixed no lefs than fix
" pieces of folid wax, perfectly white and tran-
" fparent like gum ; three upon one fide, and
" three upon the other, appearing to the eye e-
" qual in bulk and gravity ; fo that the body
" of the bee feemed duly poifed, and the flight
" not in the leaft obftructed by any inequali-
" ties.

" Here have I found it at other times, and
" once I took away eight pieces together, and I
" knew that it was wax, and nothing elfe. Will
" not this pafs for demonftration ?"

That Mr THORLEY, and probably fome o-
thers, have feen bees carrying fuch white fcales,
or pieces of folid wax, on their bodies, once
or twice perhaps in their lives, I will not dif-

pute. I myfelf have feen the fame phænomenon, once, or at moft twice, during an experience of thirty years. But it certainly would be abfurd to infer from thefe rare cafes, that all the wax, which the combs are made of, is carried into the hive in this manner. The contrary infer- ence muft be drawn, were it from nothing elfe but the confideration, that thefe white fcales have been fo very feldom obferved. It is alfo well known, that when a young fwarm is new- ly fet down, within a fhort time thereafter, fmall fcales of fine white wax will be feen on the ftool; which is a certain proof that the bees are beginning to build combs: and perhaps a few of the bees may pick up fome of thefe fcales, to prevent them from being loft. But, if every bee, that is employed in carrying wax for build- ing the combs, either within or on the outfide of her body, could be obferved, we would fee thoufands thus loaded every day after a young fwarm is firft fet down, inftead of obferving only one or two folitary inftances in the courfe of twenty or thirty years.

If a natural or artificial fwarm is confined 24 hours in a hive, after it is newly put into it, the bees will be found bufily employed in making combs. From this it may be argued,

that

that the bees, having eaten a quantity of bee
bread on purpofe, before they left their own
hive, and having it ftill in their ftomachs; had
made wax of it to erect the combs.

Of this fact any perfon may convince himfelf, by driving the bees out of any hive into
an empty one, and confining them 24 hours;
after which, upon examining the hive attentively, he will find a piece of comb, perhaps fix or
eight inches long, befides feveral hundreds of
fcales lying on the ftool. It is evident, then,
that thefe fcales could not be brought from the
field, as Mr THORLEY fuppofes, feeing the
bees were never out of the hive; and, it is farther to be obferved, that when they are at full
liberty to work in the fields, and when a young
fwarm is moft bufily employed in rearing
combs, nothing can be feen on their bodies of
thefe fcales, or any thing elfe.

I have fometimes, indeed, been inclined to
think, that the wax might be an excrefcence,
exudation, or production from the bodies of
the bees; and that, as the Queen bee can lay
eggs when fhe pleafes, if need require, fo the
working bees can produce wax from the fubftance of their own bodies. If this conjecture
be right, it will follow of courfe, that all the

food

food which the bees take, contributes to the formation of wax, in the fame manner as all the
food which a cow eats contributes to the production of milk: or, (to adopt a more near fi-
mile from the infect tribe,) as all the food
which a fpider takes, contributes not only to
the nourifhment of the animal, but to the production of the fubftance of the cob-web from its
body. Numberlefs other analogies in nature
might be adduced in favour of the probability
of this theory. The filk, for inftance, produced
from the body of the filk worm, is a fubftance as
different from that of the animal itfelf, or of the
mulberry leaf it feeds on, as wax is from that
of the body of the bee, or of the honey or flower fhe fucks. And the excrefcence produced
in the human ear, which alfo goes by the name
of *wax*, is certainly a fubftance as different
from that of the body which produces it, as
either the one or the other. Upon the whole,
until I meet with a more probable theory, fup-
ported by facts, I muft give it as my humble
opinion, that the wax is either produced from
the bodies of the bees alone, or rather that the
bees can fpeedily convert what they bring from
the flowers into it, and therewith build their
combs, and feal up both their young and their
honey.   CHAP.

C H A P. XXV.

OF THE HONEY HARVEST.

I ONCE thought, that if we preferve all our bees, we muft alfo keep all our honey in the hives, to maintain them during winter and fpring. But I am now of a different opinion; for the feverity of the winter not only reduces the number of bees, but fometimes even kills whole hives, although they have large quantities of honey in them. It is, therefore, much more profitable to preferve all the bees alive, and unite them to other hives, although we fhould be at the expence of fome honey to feed them during fpring. It is indeed, probable, that every Queen is capable of laying only a certain number of eggs. Suppofing, then, that we fhould put 100,000 common bees in a hive, the old bees would gradually die out, and as there would be but one breeding Queen in the hive, it would foon have no more bees than

any

any other hive. Indeed, experience convinces me, that there never was a hive, however large, profperous, and numerous of inhabitants in fummer, either naturally, or by being united, that did not gradually decreafe againft next fpring, fo as very little to exceed the moft ordinary hives in number. It is true, indeed, that fome fwarms of bees, by being kept in a very large hive for feveral years, have had as much honey and wax, as three or four ordinary hives. But fuch cafes only occur, either when two or three fwarms go together in fwarming time, or when a thriving fwarm continues for fome years in a large hive ; and, by collecting perhaps 60lb. of honey every year, and confuming only the half of it during winter and fpring, thus increafes the ftock of honey, and the weight of the hives, at the rate of 30lb. a-year*.

Neverthelefs

---

* I am quite certain, however, that a great number of bees in one capacious hive,—I fhall fuppofe 30,000,—will breed amazingly ; as they will have perhaps, in June or July, not under 7,000 young in the cells ; for almoft every comb in the hive at that feafon, will be quite full of eggs, nymphs and young bees, all gradually coming forward. According to this calculation, allowing 18 days to pafs between the time that an egg is laid, and a complete bee produced from it, there would not be fewer than 300 eggs laid each day in the hive,—an aftonifhing num-

be

Neverthelefs it is evident, that a hive that has a great number of bees in autumn, ftands

a

ber to be all laid by one mother. Monfieur REAUMUR fays, that the Queen will lay 200 in 24 hours ; but I am perfuaded, that, in fome extraordinarily populous hives, fhe lays near double that number. She is acknowledged by all authors to be very proli-fic. SWAMMERDANE beheld in the ovarium of a Queen bee, 5100 eggs at once ; and REAUMUR fays, that, " in the fpace of " three weeks, 6000 bees are brought to perfection." Nor, in-deed, is this at all incredible, when we confider that fome cod fifh have had no fewer than 9,344,000 eggs in their ovarium at once. * The prolific powers of the Queen bee feem to depend very much on the ftate of the hive fhe belongs to ; and I am apt to think, that the increafe of a hive fcarcely ever fails on her part, if fhe be in a healthy ftate. For, during the months of May, June, and July, all Queens breed furprifingly faft, if the weather is good, and if they have abundance of common bees to rear the young brood. When one, therefore, has a hive, that, on account of the paucity of its inhabitants, does not breed faft, were he to add a great number of common bees to it in Summer, it would foon increafe as faft as any in his apiary.

It muft, however, be allowed, that fome Queens will be more fruitful than others, although a hive feldom fuffers from that caufe alone. One fingle author alledges, that two or three Queens may be permitted to live for a fhort time in a hive, during the mid-dle of fummer, and that of courfe a greater number of eggs will be laid each day, than if there were but one Queen in the hive. But I am pretty confident, that this is a miftake ; for, among the many hundreds of fwarms, which I have driven out, I never faw more than one breeding Queen at a time. In-deed, perhaps, in one hive among fifty, I have obferved two

Queens,

* Nature delineated, p. 130.

a much better chance not to periſh by the ſeverity of the winter, than a hive that has not
half the number of inhabitants; for which
reaſon I would earneſtly recommend it to my
readers, NEVER TO KILL A SINGLE WORKING
BEE, at any ſeaſon of the year ; but, in autumn,
to unite all the bees of thoſe hives, from which
the honey is taken, to thoſe that are intended
to be kept as ſtock hives. This will render
them fit to defend themſelves both againſt the
ſeverity of the weather in winter, and againſt
robbers in ſpring ; and will alſo greatly forward their labours as ſoon as the working ſeaſon returns ; for, as has been already obſerved,
it is of the greateſt importance to have the
hives always well-ſtored with bees.

The time of taking the honey out of the
hives is ſometimes earlier, and ſometimes later,
according to the weather, and the earlineſs or
lateneſs of the flowers in the neighbourhood.

I

Queens, an old and a young one; but that hive would have ſent
off the young Queen with a new ſwarm probably in a day or
two, as ſhe was only waiting an opportunity for that purpoſe; and
it may be obſerved, that the young Queen was not then arrived at
the age of laying eggs, as ſhe is about eight days old before ſhe
can become a mother; and therefore I am fully perſuaded, that
there are never on any occaſion two Queens in the ſame hive,
laying eggs at one time.

I have known a hive of bees waste their honey,
and the hive become gradually lighter after the
first week of August; and, at other times, in
favourable weather, I have seen hives of bees,
that were situated near heath, (as mentioned,
page 185) continue working keenly during the
whole of August, and the greater part of September, and become daily heavier. In a word,
the harvest of honey, like that of corn, is earlier or later, more plentiful or scarce, in different years, according to the weather and the climate, and the variety of seasons and situations.

One general rule, however, may be laid
down for the proper time to take honey. As
soon as the flowers, in the neighbourhood of
an apiary, are mostly faded, although the bees
may continue to work in favourable days, yet
their families being now generally very large,
they will probably consume as much honey in
one day, as they will collect in two. At this
period, therefore, the prudent bee-master will
first choose his stock hives, according to the directions given, page 89. He will then put a
mark on every hive he has picked out for this
purpose, and sell or take the honey from all the
rest, whether good or bad; for the sooner the
honey is taken, it will run the more easily out

C c   of

of the combs. And, as it runs beſt in warm weather, he ſhould take the honey, that he intends to run out of the combs, immediately after the bees have nearly given over work, and unite the bees to his ſtock hives, as directed page 136, &c.

But honey, that is intended to be kept in the combs, ought not to be taken ſo ſoon, as cold weather renders the combs more fit to be handled ; and as the bees are all to be kept alive, and of courſe muſt be maintained, it is of no conſequence, in point of expence, whether they are allowed to feed on the honey in the hive they are ſoon to leave, or on that of the hive to which they are to be united. Beſides, there is an additional advantage, that ariſes from their being allowed to continue in their native hive ; as the longer they remain in it, the more young bees will be hatched ; which both preſerves a greater number of bees, and makes the honey combs more free of the young brood ; ſo that there is no harm in keeping the bees in the hives till October, when the honey is not intended to be run out of them.

When the honey of a hive is taken in Autumn, and there is a great number of young in the cells, thoſe combs which contain the young,

and

and which may be intermingled with bee-bread, ſhould be carefully and gently placed in an eek, (ſee page 110, &c.), and a numerous hive put over it, to hatch out the young brood, and ſuck up the particles of honey remaining in the combs, and probably alſo make ſome uſe of the bee-bread. This plan is of great advantage to the bee-maſter, as the young bees, which are always the beſt, and which would otherwiſe have been totally loſt, will thus be all pre-ſerved; beſides that very little uſe could have been made of ſuch honey in the cells, as was mixed with young bees, eggs, and bee-bread. The eek and the combs may be removed in a-bout three or four weeks thereafter, and the hive ſet down in its former ſtation.

If the bee-maſter has not as many good hives as he wiſhes to keep for ſtock, he may ſup-ply himſelf, by conjoining the bees and honey of two light hives, and uniting them into one in September, as mentioned in page 47. The hea-vieſt hive ſhould be firſt ſelected; after which, the bees and honey ſhould be taken out of the light hives in the following manner:

The Bee-maſter muſt firſt drive as many of the bees as poſſible into an empty hive, as di-

reſted

rected in page 138. But, at this period, and in all cold feafons, bees are not fo eafily driven out as in warm weather; although, the taking them into a warm room, will make them run up the better. Afterwards, he fhould take the combs carefully out, efpecially if it be a light young hive, one by one, with his hand; and, in doing this, all the bees that are upon the combs may be gently fwept off with a large feather, into the hive, among their brethren. Their Queen muft then be taken away, with a-bout 100 bees, and kept clofe prifoners; then re-inforce any hive with the common bees that appears to have feweft inhabitants in it, (as directed p. 136, &c.) or rather any hive that will give them the moft favourable reception; and, as foon as all the bees are united and happy, the Queen, with her hundred attendants, may be introduced; and, if they judge her to be preferable to their own, (for the bees are doubt-lefs the beft judges in thefe matters) perhaps they will elect her and banifh their own Queen. About two days thereafter, the hive intended for the ftock may be re-inforced with the honey combs; according to the directions given in pages 110, 111, and 112.

The Bee-mafter fhould proceed in the fame

manner

manner with every other hive, from which he
intends to take honey ; and if any of his neighbours ſhould happen to be ſtill ſo prejudiced in
favour of old cuſtoms, as to continue the barbarous practice of killing their bees, he may
make an advantageous bargain with them, and
ſave the lives of the uſeful inſects, by offering
a trifle for them, which will ſurely be accepted,
as the owners can otherwiſe gain nothing by
them. By uniting theſe to his own hives, every hive in his apiary will be fully ſupplied with
bees and honey : And being now in a proſpe-
rous ſtate, may be carefully covered over, and
rendered fit to endure the winter. See page 97.

C H A P. XXVI.

OF PREPARING HONEY AND WAX.

Before entering upon this neceſſary buſineſs,
the bee-maſter ſhould be properly provided
with a ſufficient number of utenſils, ſuch as
large diſhes, jars, ſieves, knives and ſpoons.
He ſhould begin while the honey is warm, as
it

it will run from the combs the more quickly;
and therefore, to preferve the heat till the operation is over, the hive fhould be brought into
a warm room. ·He fhould next take hold of
the ends of the crofs fticks in the hive with
pincers, and loofen them by twifting them
round; after which they will be eafily pulled
out. The edges of the combs fhould then be
loofened with a knife from the hive all around.
Upon giving the hive a gentle knock on the
floor, on that fide which is oppofite to the
broad fide of the combs, they will fall to that
fide, and upon turning the hive, and giving it
another knock on the oppofite fide, all the
combs, which could be reached by the knife
will be effectually loofened. The hive being
ftill kept on its broad fide, the combs will all
be above each other. The uppermoft being
firft taken off, if there are any dead bees in it,
they may be blown or brufhed off. The combs
fhould then be divided into three parts. The
empty combs being firft laid afide for wax;
next the combs containing eggs or maggots;
and laftly, the moft valuable part of the whole,
the fine fealed combs, containing the honey,
fhould be laid in a veffel by themfelves. An
affiftant fhould immediately be ordered to cut

thefe

thefe laft into thin flices, firft obferving to pare off the fealed mouths of the cells, that the honey may run freely out. In this ftate they fhould be laid in fieves, or any other veffels that will afford a free paffage to the honey, which will run quite clear, and the honey thus obtained fhould be kept by itfelf, as being the pureft and beft.

Thofe combs which may be filled with a mixture of live young maggots, bee-bread and honey, fhould immediately * be put below ftock hives, as directed page 202, &c. and the bees will foon fuck up all the honey in them. When the fine combs are completely run, they fhould be put into a pan, over a flow fire, and ftirred conftantly till they are more than milk warm; when they fhould be put into a ftrong canvafs bag, and the honey fqueezed out. This honey being of an inferior quality, may be either ufed in the family, for common ufes; or rather kept for feeding the bees. All the combs, from which it was fqueezed, may then be foaked in water, and a weak kind of mead

---

* All combs containing eggs and young in the cells muft be put immediately to other hives, while they are warm; for, fhould they remain two or three hours out of a hive, they will become chill and cool, fo as to make them decay in the cells.

mead drawn from them; or a ftronger mead may be taken from the combs by foaking them, after the fineft of the honey is run off, without melting or fqueezing them at all. Indeed, in warm weather, fine combs will run almoft quite dry, without the leaft preffure.

My method of running honey is this : I hang up a wide riddle, with the fliced honey combs in it, about 5 feet from the ground : About 8 or 10 inches below this, I place a fieve, fomewhat wider in circumference than the riddle, and, at an equal diftance under the fieve, a fine fearch, proportionally wider than the fieve, under which, a foot lower ftill, I place one of my earthen covers, defcribed page 98, with the bottom uppermoft, and a fmall hole in the top, to anfwer the purpofe of a funnel. This laft being properly fixed in a veffel of a fufficient fize, the honey that runs into it is completely purified from all extraneous matter whatever, by running through fo many different fieves at one time. Thus, in a few hours, in a warm day, I can have my honey purified to the higheft degree of finenefs, without boiling or diluting it, or ufing any other means that would deprive it of its original genuine flavour ; for any fmall crumbs of wax, bee-bread or the like, that pafs through

the

the riddle, are caught by the fieve; and if any thing ftill fmaller fhould pafs through the fieve, it is intercepted by the fearch, which permits nothing but the pureft honey to pafs through the funnel into the receiving veffel; and thus the whole procefs is completed in a fhort time. During this procefs, the combs in the riddle may now and then be turned over with a knife, to make the honey run the more freely.

This method fhould be adopted by all Bee-mafters, who have many hives and much honey to run. But fuch as have but a fmall quantity may follow the other plan, and their honey will do very well, if they only keep it free of young bees and bee-bread : for a few crumbs of wax running through the fieve will not hurt the honey, as it will foon rife to the furface, and can be eafily fkimmed off.

The combs being now entirely free of honey, the next operation neceffary is to make wax. My method of performing this is quite fimple. I boil the combs in a kettle, with a fufficient quantity of water, over a flow fire, for about 40 minutes, during which time they are all melted, and I ftir them about frequently all the time. I then take two or three ladle-fulls, and put into a bag, fewed together in

D d the

the form of a funnel, and which is commonly
called *Hippocrates's Lever.* It is made of thin
strong canvass, and of such a length, that the
upper part may come over the end of a board,
which leans upon my breast, while the other
end of it is placed in a vessel fit to receive
the wax, from which I press out the water and
the wax, pretty much in the same way that the
tanners dress their leather.

I generally boil what remains in the bag a
second time, and squeeze it again to obtain
more wax. By this method, however, the wax
cannot be got entirely out of the drofs; nor indeed can it be obtained by any other mode that
I have ever seen or heard of being attempted.
All the wax that is ultimately left among the
drofs, in this way of separating it, is of very
little value, and would not refund the expence
of any further trouble. *

After the wax is cooled in the tub, I again
put it into the kettle with clean water, and having

ing

* I have tried several other methods, in order to extract all the
wax from the drofs. Near twenty years ago, I got a press made
for this purpose, somewhat resembling those which the candle-
makers use to squeeze their tallow with; but, finding it did not
answer the purpose, I laid it aside. I have also put in practice
Mr Keys's method, but, after repeated trials, found it not satis-
factory.

ing melted it, I pour it into a bowl or veffel, ‡ which is wider at the top than at the
bottom, and fkim off any drofs that may float
on the top of the wax. After allowing it to
ftand in fome warm place, that it may cool gradually, which prevents it from cracking, I take
out the cake of wax, and pare off all the drofs
from the under fide, till there be nothing
left but what is fit for the merchant. The
fkimmings and parings fhould be kept and
boiled over again, next time any more wax is
made, in order to obtain as much wax as poffible.

‡ A veffel made fomething like a flower pot, that is both narrow and deep, anfwers beft for this purpofe : as the good wax
rifes to the top, and the droffy part is much more eafily feparated
from it, than when the veffel is broad and fhallow ; as in this
cafe, the cake of wax is thin, and not fo eafily feparated from the
drofs, when cold.

CHAP.

CHAP. XXVII.

OF THE DIFFERENT KINDS OF HONEY.

I⊤ appears that honey does not candy from cold alone, without fome other concurring circumftances ; for among a number of hives, all equally expofed to the fame degree of cold, fome will be found to have candied honey in them, while others have none. Even in the fame hive, a comb will fometimes be found, with honey in it, partly candied and partly liquid : And it is well known, that fome honey will turn thick and candy, almoft as foon as it is run out of the cells, fo early as the month of Auguft ; while other honey will continue liquid till November, December, or January : And fome very fine honey will remain till April, before it candy. From all thefe facts, it muft be inferred, that there are other concurring circumftances befides cold, that co-operate with it in occafioning honey to candy. What thefe circumftances are, it is difficult to determine.

mine. My opinion is, that the candying of honey proceeds partly from the nature of the flowers from which it is collected, and partly from the time that it has remained in the hive. But againſt this laſt ſuppoſition an objection ariſes, from this conſideration, that the very fineſt of what is called *virgin honey*, will ſome-times candy very ſoon after it has run from the combs, and become like fine white ſugar *.

This fine white honey is collected from white clover, and alſo from ſome other flowers which yield a white juice, and it is reckoned by moſt people the fineſt of honey. But the ſpecies of honey which continues longeſt in a liquid ſtate, and

---

* Many authors affirm, that honey, candied in the comb, is ve-ry deſtructive to bees, and alledge, that they may as well eat poiſon; others inſiſt, that it chokes them; while a third claſs alledge, that it hurts them by bedaubing them, with many o-ther whimſical ſuppoſitions. But theſe authors certainly have either taken their own dreams for realities, or have wrote upon truſt; which they certainly ought not, in a caſe that can be ſo eaſily decided by experiment. For let any perſon put a piece of comb into a hive, with the honey in the cells, partly candied and partly liquid, and he will find, that the bees will ſoon ſuck up all the liquid honey in the upper parts of the cells; and if the middle part of the honey be candied, they will throw it out, and thus get at the liquid honey in the under parts;—which they will chearfully feed upon, without either choking, bedaub-ing, or poiſoning themſelves with it, and rejoice that they have got ſo much proviſion at ſo little expence of time and labour.

and is efteemed by many connoiffeurs the very beft of honey, (as it undoubtedly is as good
as any,) is of a flightly greenifh colour, and is
likewife collected from white flowers. When
candied, it fometimes confifts of fine white particles, refembling fmall hail, intermixed with
fome liquid honey, and is very beautiful.

Heath produces a fine high-coloured honey,
which looks alfo very beautiful in the virgin
comb, fhining like gold through the pure tranfparent cells. The gentlemen and ladies about
Newcaftle are very fond of this kind of honey in
the combs. When run into pots and candied,
it becomes all hard and griftly,—a fpecies
of honey which is alfo greatly efteemed by
many.

There is another kind of honey, which is collected from all the above-mentioned flowers,
and which, having been kept two or three years
in the hive, is therefore called *old honey.* Some
of that kind of honey will be very fine tafted,
and pretty griftly when eat, but the greateft
part of it, when it is run out of the combs,
becomes in a few days thereafter thick and
fmooth ; and is, on that account, fufpected, by
people who are ignorant of the nature of honey, to have been adulterated, and mixed up
                                        with

with butter, fugar, flower, and the like. This miftake prevails in many parts of the country, and it is much to be regretted ; as this fufpicion, fo injurious to the charaĉters of honeft country people, who, in reality, fell their honey as it run from the combs, is even fometimes entertained by perfons in the higher ranks of life, who might be expected to be better informed. For although the country dealers fometimes fpoil their honey, by fqueezing out the combs, and ·thereby occafioning bee-bread, eggs, &c. to mingle with it ; yet in all my experience, I have never met with any honey, which I could difcover to have been mixed with butter, fugar or flour. Once indeed, and only once, I faw honey which the owner had mixed with water, but he was juftly punifhed for his avarice ; for the honey and water, fomented by the carriage in fuch a manner, that the upper part of it had more the appearance of barm or yeft than of honey ; and the unfortunate dealer loft both his cargo and his charaĉter.

Some alledge, that honey may be purified by warming or boiling it in pots, &c. which occafions it to throw up a fcum, that is fkimmed off. But I am perfuaded, that honey is always beft in its natural ftate ; and that fuch methods

of

of refining it, inftead of improving the honey, often communicate a bad tafte or flavour to it. I therefore ufe no other method with my honey, than to let it run freely from the combs, as above, and take particular care, that none of the eggs or bee-bread, get amongft it. And indeed this is all the art which is required to make the very fineft of honey ;—namely, cleanlinefs : Let it only be keep as clean as the bees kept it, and the fineft of honey will be the produce.

C H A P. XXVIII.

OF THE VARIOUS ENEMIES OF BEES, AND HOW TO GUARD
AGAINST THEM.

O̶F all the enemies the bees have hitherto had to encounter, MAN may juftly be confidered as the greateft. For while he follows the old barbarous cuftom of killing whole hives of that induftrious race, for the fake of their honey, (a cuftom which, in many nations, has begun to yield to a more œconomical, as well as a more

humane

humane practice,) he certainly deſtroys more
of theſe his faithful ſervants, annually, than a-
ny other claſs of animals whatever, or, indeed,
than all the other beaſts, birds, and inſects u-
nited, ever did. Nor are thoſe prejudiced mur-
derers of the bees, their only enemies among
mankind. The predatory claſs, who ſteal either their honey, or the whole hives, prove e-
qually deſtructive to them. But it is to be hop-
ed, that as ſelf intereſt and humanity equally
unite in exploding the practice of the murder-
ers, ſo the effectual execution of the laws will
prove a ſufficient protection from the thieves †.

The three next greateſt enemies of the bees
are, Cold, Famine, and Robbers of their own
ſpecies: To which may be added, as the fourth
moſt deſtructive claſs of enemies, mice. By
one or other of theſe, or all of them united,
hundreds of hives of bees periſh annually in
Britain, while their other enemies hurt them
but rarely or partially.

E e   Of

---

† Perhaps I can boaſt of a degree of good fortune, in this reſpect, that ſcarcely one in the kingdom can equal; for, notwithſtanding the great number of bee-hives I have had ſtanding in the
midſt of muirs, and far from any houſes, I never had a ſingle hive
ſtolen but one, nor ever loſt one ſingle ſwarm to my knowledge,
by their flying away in ſwarming time:

Of the former, we need say nothing here, having already given sufficient directions in the preceding part of this work, how to guard against cold, famine, robbers, and mice; and shall, therefore, proceed to point out some of the latter.

WASPS are great enemies to bees, especially in warm dry years; and those hives that are near plantations, where they often resort, are the greatest sufferers by them. In my neighbourhood, wasps are seldom very troublesome, except that sometimes a mother wasp will appear before a hive in May, and offer to go in; but her hoarse voice and strange dress soon discover her to the bees, who banish her from their habitation. I know not if any hive in my neighbourhood was ever much hurt by wasps; but, a few miles distant from this, sundry hives have been sometimes considerably the worse of them.

The best way to extirpate wasps is to destroy their Queen or mother, in spring, wherever she can be found; for wasps, in this respect, as well as in some other particulars, resemble bees; and therefore, when a mother wasp is killed, a whole nest of them is in effect destroyed. Their nests, however, should also be carefully sought out,

and

and as many of them deftroyed as poffible, by
burning, fcalding, or drowning them; left, like
the bees, the wafps fhould alfo poffefs the power of raifing a Queen mother from a common
egg.

When a number of wafps attempt to enter a-
ny, hive about the end of fummer or beginning
of autumn, the entry fhould be reduced to half
an inch in length, and fcarce as much in height,
that the bees may be able to defend it; and thofe
hives that have but few bees in them fhould be
taken, and their bees united to other hives, as
directed page 141, &c. But fuch as are intended for ftock hives, if feverely attacked by wafps,
fhould be removed to fome fituation diftant
from plantations, and kept there, till the feafon
of plundering, by both wafps and bees, is over.
Veffels may alfo be placed in the apiary, with
honey or fugar in them mixed with ale, which
will allure and deftroy the wafps; but in fine
days thefe veffels fhould be removed, left they
fhould likewife allure and deftroy the bees. A-
nother difadvantage alfo frequently attends this
method of deftroying the wafps; as thefe veffels,
placed in apiaries, are apt to attract all the wafps
in the neighbourhood, and thus, by bringing
hundreds that would not otherwife have come,

render

render the remedy worfe than the difeafe. This
fhould, therefore, be cautioufly avoided; and
indeed, in general, this method is of no great
fervice.

The large moth, called the WAX MOTH, from
its maggots feeding on the wax, is another
great enemy of the bees. This animal is extremely alert at difcovering any crevice, about
the outfide of the fkirts of the hive, to depofit
her eggs in; and when unfuccefsful in fuch
attempts, fhe nimbly runs in at the entry, un-
perceived by the bees, and.lays her eggs, which
quickly become large white maggots, above
half an inch each in length. Thefe maggots
fpin over themfelves a covering for their defence, and become very numerous in fome
hives. Their depredations difcourage the bees
fo much, that they fometimes defert the hive.

For my own part, I never fuffered the fmalleft lofs by thefe invaders: I never faw one of
their maggots in any of my hives, except twice
or thrice, that I obferved a few of them in one
hive; and I never heard any bee-mafter in my
neighbourhood complain of them. But, a-
bout twenty miles diftant, I once faw a dozen
of wax moths in one hive; and the owner told
me, that he had once two hives in one feafon,
which

which had as many of thefe moth maggots in them as bees; for which reafon he burnt them both, with their bees, combs, honey, wax moths and maggots altogether. In doing this he thought he acted prudently; but, in my o-pinion, he would have acted a much wifer part, if he had driven all the bees that were in them, into empty hives and made two fwarms of them, or re-inforced weak hives, with them; and then fmoaked the wax moths and mag-gots to death: after which, he might have given the bees of his other hives the combs to fuck the honey from them, and then melted the wax. His empty hive could have ferved another year, and thus he would have fuffered no lofs whatever, except that of the young bees, which would have been very trifling in com-parifon of lofing all. The pooreft and weakeft hives are moft infefted with wax moths, as well as with other enemies. When any figns of fuch vermin appear, either without or within a hive, they fhould be inftantly deftroyed.

Birds of different kinds are alfo enemies to bees; efpecially in Spring, when they catch them on purpofe to feed their young with; fuch as the fwallow, the fparrow, the lark, the duck, and even the common hen. I myfelf have

feen

feen hens pick up bees ; but they very feldom hurt them much. Birds, in general, however, ought to be guarded againft by all poffible means. A fcare-crow placed near a hive will fometimes frighten away the wild birds.

SPIDERS likewife deftroy fome bees by catching them in their nets and fucking their blood; though a ftrong bee will fometimes break through the flimfy texture, and efcape. Nothing is eafier than to protect them from this enemy, by deftroying the cob-webs as foon as they appear about the hives, or their ftools or covers.

EARWIGS are alfo formidable enemies to bees ; and Mr Keys fays, that " they fteal into " the hive at night and drag out bee after bee, " fucking out their vitals, and leaving nothing " but their fkins, like fo many fcalps or trophies " of their butchery." They breed between the fkirts of the hive and the ftool, where their nefts ought to be fearched for and deftroyed.

" ANTS, (fays Mr WILDMAN,) fometimes " make their nefts between the hive and the " covering, without molefting the bees or be- " ing molefted." Although, for my own part, I was never fenfible of my bees receiving any

injury

injury from ants, yet I have heard ſome bee-
maſters ſay, that they go into hives during the
night, and ſuck the honey; and that they
have ſeen hives ruined by them. To guard
againſt ſuch poſſible depredations, the covers
ſhould be now and then removed, in the end of
Summer, and the ants deſtroyed.

WOOD-LICE are alſo hurtful to bees. When
old decayed wood, which they harbour in,
happens to be near a hive, either the wood ſhould
be removed to a diſtance, or the wood-lice
carefully ſearched for and extirpated.

BAD WEATHER, wind, rain, and the ex-
tremes of cold and heat, &c. have already
been repeatedly noticed as prejudicial to bees,
and may be guarded againſt by the ſituations
of the apiaries, covering the hives properly, &c.

NOISE is alſo ſomewhat hurtful to bees, as
it diſturbs them in their induſtrious operations. This can likewiſe be in general eaſily
prevented, by placing the hives in a quiet ſi-
tuation, remote from noiſy operations, high
ways and the like.

To conclude,—FILTH and IMPURITY of e-
very kind that may gather upon the ſtool, or a-
round the outſide of the hive, or be introduced
near the hive, ſo as to occaſion diſagreeable
effluvia,

effluvia, ought to be carefully removed and
guarded againſt, by keeping the hives and e-
very thing near them perfectly ſweet and
clean.

C H A P. XXIX.

CONCLUSION.

As the principal intention of this work is to
ſtimulate the attention of the public towards
an important object, that has been hitherto
too much neglected, I ſhall conclude with a
few words of advice to people of all ranks and
degrees amongſt us, on the ſubject.

And, *firſt*, I would humbly advife all GEN-
TLEMEN OF LANDED PROPERTY, to conſider,
whether they have not multitudes of mellifluous
flowers growing in many places of their grounds,
which might yield annually ſeveral hundred
pints of honey, as well as many pounds of wax,
with very little trouble or expence, but whoſe
ſweets being overlooked and neglected, ſerve
only to feed the caterpillars and the waſps.

In

In the next place, I would serioufly advife every CLERGYMAN, whether belonging to the e-ftablished church, or to any other sect or party, to keep a few bee hives in his garden, or upon his glebe. I have for feveral years past paid a clergyman's lady in my neighbourhood fome pounds for honey and wax, which she had to fpare after her own family was ferved. I have, in my poffeffion, two books on the fubject of bees, wrote by two clergymen, one of whom had EIGHTY SIX fwarms in one year.

Mr Wheeler likewife informs us, that while he was viewing the beauties of Parnaffus, he was entertained by a clergyman with the fweets of a repaft of honey. " After I had difcourfed " fome time," fays he †, " with the good old " Caloyer, (Prieft) whom they efteemed a Saint, I " was conducted into a garden well planted with " beans and peas, (this was at the end of Janu- " ary,) and another by it, furnished with four " or five hundred ftocks of bees. The good old " Caloyer prefently went, took a ftock of bees, " and brought me a little of delicate white ho- " ney combs, with bread and olives, and very

F f " good

---

† A Journey into Greece, by George Wheeler, Efq; in com-pany with Dr Spon of Lyons, p. 411.

" good wine; to which he set us down in his
" hut, and made us a dinner, with far greater
" satisfaction than the most princely banquet
" in Europe could have afforded us."

That the number of our hives might be
greatly increased, wherever there is proper pasture for bees, appears evidently from Mr Wheeler's narrative, and is confirmed by the following passage in the account lately published of
the sheep in Spain.

" If sheep loved aromatic plants, it would be
" one of the greatest misfortunes that could be-
" fal the farmers in Spain. The number of
" bee-hives there is incredible. I am almost
" ashamed to give under my hand, that I knew
" a parish priest who had five thousand hives."

GENTLEMEN FARMERS ought, therefore, by
no means to neglect the culture of bees. They
have almost as many advantages as the proprietors themselves. The great quantities of clover,
mustard, and heath, with which their grounds
in general abound, would maintain a bee-hive
for every horse and cow they have upon their
grounds. And gentlemen STORE-MASTERS
might keep at least a couple of hives for every
score of sheep they have in their sheep-walks.
Indeed, farmers of every rank will find their
                                        advantage

advantage in keeping bee-hives, in proportion to the extent of the flowers that grow upon their farms; as one fingle acre, planted with turnips, muftard, clover, or heath, will feed many hives. Even the meaneft cottager, who has but a cottage and a kail-yard, might keep two or three hives, and fow a little muftard and turnips, or plant a few goofeberry bufhes, on purpofe to feed his bees. There is fcarce a country village in the kingdom, that might not afford to keep as many bee-hives as there are dwelling houfes in it; nor a tradefman in fuch a village, who might not eafily keep as many hives as he has hands employed in his bufinefs. Even fervants might have a few hives kept as their own property, in the gardens of their parents, brothers, or friends. In fhort, perfons of all ranks and degrees, from the KING to the cottager, might be profitably employed, or agreeably amufed, by keeping bee-hives †.

F f 2   Let

---

† I am quite certain, and fome others have often told me, that they were of the fame opinion, that the melodious humming of bees, when bufy at work, or fporting in the air for their own amufement, will have fuch an effect upon the animal fpirits, that, however chagrined or ruffled the temper of a perfon might be, before he takes a walk among his bees, he generally does not withdraw till the mind enjoys a perfect calm and inward tranquillity.

Let none here alledge, that thefe our induftrious infects are below the attention of the
greateft. MELISSUS, the firft inventor of bee-
hives, was a king ; but perhaps we fhould never
have heard of him, if he had not paid particular attention to thefe his little fubjects. Encouragement might alfo be given to the culture of
bees, by refpectable focieties, fuch as the Board
of Agriculture, the Highland Society, &c. who
might advertife fmall premiums, to be given
to thofe who fhould rear the greateft number of hives, or bring the greateft quantity of
honey and wax to the market during the feafon. Perfons properly qualified might alfo be
employed, either by focieties or individuals, to
infpect the ftate of the hives within certain dif-
tricts. One perfon, thus employed by a fociety,
might overfee all the hives within two or three
counties in one feafon ; correcting, as he went a-
long, whatever he found amifs either in the ftate
or in the management of them, and ftrictly en-
joining, that not a fingle bee fhould be killed at
any feafon of the year. The increafe of bee-
hives might alfo be rapidly forwarded, if proprietors of ground, upon giving leafes to their
tenants, were to make it an article in their tack,
that the tenant fhould furnifh the proprietor
with fo many pints of honey produced upon
                                                    his

his own ground, annually, in proportion to the situation and extent of his farm, and for which he should be allowed the highest market price. And hints might be occasionally given in the newspapers, calling the attention of the public to perform the necessary offices about their bees, at the proper seasons of the year ; as well as to inform the world when any new discovery of their nature, or improvement in their management, happens to be made.

Thus I have laid down a PLAN, in terms plain and intellegible to every capacity, for INCREASING THE NUMBER OF BEE-HIVES IN SCOTLAND ; and have showed how HONEY and WAX may be increased to a PRODIGIOUS A-MOUNT, by a proper exertion upon the part of all who have any favourable situations for hives, but especially of gentlemen of property, who must be supposed to have the greatest variety of such advantages. And I now take farewell of my readers, by assuring them, upon the credit of near THIRTY YEARS EXPERIENCE, that the plan I have laid down is no chimæra, or *Will-o'-the-wisp*, but that, by strictly adhering to the preceding directions, they may depend upon meeting with the utmost success.

FINIS.

INDEX.

INDEX,

A

G g   weather,

Cases

E.

Eel,

Famine,

F

Famine, directions to preserve bees from, 110, 115, 131 ; *see* Food.

Farmers, gentlemen, advised to rear bees, 226, 227.

Feeding, see Combs, and Food.

Filth hurtful to bees, 223, 224.

Flowers, melifluous, the number of, in Britain almost infinite, vi. ; the principal ones proper for bees, catalogue of, 11, 13, 14, 15 ; no kind of, refused by them, 16 ; those first pitched on, preferred ever after, *ib. ;* honey contained in all flowers, 23 ; thousands of millions of them in Scotland, 33, 34 ; artificial to be raised, where natural ones fail, 40 ; various kinds recommended to be sown, 43, 44 : bees fly far in search of, 44, 45.

Food, directions how to supply bees with, 110 ; four methods, 111, 113, 114, 115 ; weight of those hives that need supplies, 125, 126 ; a hive with few bees will generally require none, 126 ; bees should be fed, when young drones are torn out before swarming, 183 ; feeding combs should be placed before hives whose situations are changed, 187.

Frozen bees, method to recover, 106.

Furze, the flowers of, grateful to bees, 15 ; blossoms early and continues long in flower, *ib.* ; advantage of rearing, 40 ; ought to be sown on dykes or waste ground, 43.

G

Geddie, John, Esq; a writer on bees, 2 ; the inventor of colony hives, 147.

Generation of bees, a mistake concerning the, 2.

Gentleman, opinion of an intelligent, respecting the change of syrup into honey, 22, 23 ; his experiment in proof of this, 23 ; anecdote of another, 44.

Gentlemen of property, the increase of Bee-hives begin to occupy the attention of, 26 ; called upon to exert themselves,

27,

H.

H h *Highland*

Honey,

INDEX.

sifted in this work, 182; their manner of killing the drones, *ib.*; the author's manner, 183, 184; *see* Drones.

L.

Lammas, the situations of bees should be changed about, 185.

Law, said to be against allowing dead hives to stand in apiaries, 157; if not, it should be enacted, *ib.*; an erroneous decision on this subject, *ib.*; would be a bad precedent, 158: no person would be sure of his swarms, *ib.*; difficulty stated, *ib.*, solved, *ib.*

Leases, a hint respecting the granting of, to tenants, 228.

Lime, plaster, the skirts of hives should be closed up with, and the entries straitened, 96.

Loaded bees, time when they begin to appear, 132; at first can be easily counted, 133; in the heat of summer, defy all power of numeration, *ib.* *see* Bees, Hives, &c.

London, the author went from Berwick to, in order to converse with Mr Wildman about bees, v; could carry an hundred bee-hives to, 140.

Lying-out hive, how to treat a, 176; *see* Hives, Swarming.

M.

Maggots, decayed, found in hives, 128; *see* Hives.

Man, hitherto the chief enemy of bees, 216, 217.

Management of bees, directions for the, in winter, 99, *et seq.* in March, April, and May, 121, *et seq.*, *see* Bees, Cold, Hives, &c.

March, bees begin to carry loads in, 125; directions how to manage bees in, 121, & *seq.* *see* Bees, Hives, &c.

Maxwell, R. a writer on bees, 2; quoted, 157.

May, how to manage bees in, 121, & *seq.* particular attention to be paid to bees this month, 131; how to choose a hive at this period, 134; *see* Bees, Hives, Management, &c.

Mead, a substitute for ale and porter, 41; may be made
weak

O.

Oak, the leaves of, honey dew found on, 18, 19.

Oeconomy rural, the culture of bees a branch of, within the reach of the poorest cottager, vii.

Old people, the increase of bee hives would afford employment for, 48, 49, 150.

Order and regularity great among bees, 53.

Over-stocking fields with bees, no danger of, 34, 35, 36.

Oziers, the flowers of, afford honey and work for bees, 15.

P.

Parnassus, account of a repast of honey at, 225.

Parishes, some, that have not twenty hives, might maintain three hundred, 32; a thousand hives in each would not extract the half of the honey in their flowers, 37.

Parliament, an act of, should be passed, if no law already exists, against allowing dead hives to remain in apiaries, 157.

Pasturage of bees, ii. *see* Flowers, Mustard, Rape, &c.

Pasture, good, bees thrive best near, 10.

Patriots called upon to attend to the subject of this treatise, 27.

Paucity of bee-hives, reasons for the, in Scotland, 28, 29, 30.

Philiscus, a contemplator of bees, 2.

Philosophers puzzled to account for the diversity of talents among mankind, iii.; antient, who contemplated bees, 1. 2, 144; bees worthy the attention of, 3; colony hives useful to the inquisitive, 147.

Plane-trees, the flowers of, afford food for bees, 13; highly agreeable to them, *ib.*; ought to be planted on purpose, 43.

Pleasure of keeping bees; 1, 3; of the bee-master in seeing his hives swarming, 151, 152; *see* Bees, Hives, &c.

Poetical eulogium on bees, 7; picture of their wars, 117.

Poland, a market for purchasing bees cheap, 49.

Poor among mankind, bees resemble the, 16; the culture of bees would afford employment for, 48, 49.

Poor

O.

fupernumerary

R.

Rat:

Rape, one of the principal plants that produce flowers proper for bees, 11, 13 ; flowers later than turnips, 13.

Reasons for the paucity of bee-hives in Scotland, 28, 29, 30, 31 ; for increasing their number, 32.

Reaumur, a writer on bees, quoted, 191, 199.

Re-inforcing bee-hives, directions for, 135, *et seq.* definition and object of, 136 ; circumstances that render it necessary, *ib. ;* precautions, *ib.* ; ambassadors should be sent to the deficient hive, 137. bees will fight at one time and unite at another, 138 ; driving and rapping described, *ib.* 139 ; the operation quite easy, 140 ; how to re-inforce weak hives, 141, 142, 143.

Remedies for the sting of a bee, 87, 88.

Removing of bee-hives, 91, from a great distance by land, 92 ; danger of jolting, 93 ; water carriage far preferable, 94.

Rich proprietors advised to raise turnips, 12 ; might make much more of their bees than they do, 30.

Robberies and wars of bees, 116 ; described, 117 ; danger of coming near the battle, *ib. ;* causes, 118 ; how to distinguish robbers, 119 ; and get rid of them, *ib.* 120 ; robbers of the human species destructive to bees, 217 ; as well as those of their own, *ib.*

Roguish bee-masters, dead hives left by, to entice their neighbours swarms, 157 ; ought to be strictly punished, *ib. ;* (*see* Law) a roguish honey dealer justly rewarded, 215.

Royal cells erected to rear Queens, 60, *see* Cells.

Runches, the flowers of, proper food for bees, 13.

Russia, bees might be imported cheap from, 49 ; endure a severe cold in, 105 ; the cold as great here one week lately, as in, 106.

S

Safe-guard, or harness, described, 83.

Sallows, the flowers of, afford work and materials for bees, 15 ; ought to be planted by men of property, 43.

Samson's dead lion, made a hive of, by the bees, 148.

Sauvages, Abbe Boiffier de, his teftimony that ants fip honey
dew, 19.

Scales, fmall white, of wax, defcribed, 192 ; Mr Thorley's account of them, *ib.* 193 ; very feldom feen, 193, 194 ; his
inferences as to the formation of wax, controverted, *ib.* ;
and refuted, 194, 195.

Schirach, Mr, refutes fome old errors refpecting the Queen bee
and drones, 53, 54 ; his experiments fatisfactory, 54.

Scotland, conjecture refpecting the quantity of honey and wax
it might produce, 23, 24 ; reafons why there are fo few
bee-hives in it, 28, 29 ; probability that bees were formerly more plentifull in it, *ib.* ; abundantly fupplied with proper food for bees, 32, 33, 34.

Screens, in exceffive hot weather, fhould be ufed to keep off the
fun's rays, 155.

Seafons, the worft, a tolerable quantity of honey produced in,
viii.

September, how to choofe ftock hives in, 88 ; the Bee-mafter's
feed time and harveft, 89 ; hives cheapeft then, *ib. fee* Hives.

Siberia, the cold in Scotland for one week, laft winter, as great
as in, 106.

Sinclair, Sir John, the author's firft meeting with, x. the fortunate confequences, *ib.* xi. xii. *fee* Author.

Situations, unfavourable for bees, 35 ; fuch as are proper for
bee-hives, numerous in Scotland, 40 ; early, recommended,
124 ; advantages of changing them, to better pafturage,
185, *& feq.* the only danger, 186 ; directions how to
change them, *ib.* ; how long to keep the bees prifoners,
ib. ; and how to treat them, 187 ; the removal fhould be to
fome diftance, *ib.* ; bad confequences if too near, 188,
189.

Snails, the whole genus of, faid to be hermaphrodites, 66 ; often creep into hives. 97 ; but feldom do much hurt *ib*

Society, the Highland, the author receives a Premium from, xi.
fee Highland.

Soliloquy in a garden, 33, 34.

Song of the bees, a fign of their health, 102.

Spain

tween

tween the Queens, 174; how to act when half the young
fwarm have been prevented from emigrating, 175; with
a fmall fwarm and lying-out hive, 176; with two fmall
fwarms, 177; with an old hive that has a royal cell, and
an empty one, *ib.*; with a hive that has long lien out,
178; the author's former practice, *ib.*; now almoft entirely given up, 179; how to return a fwarm, when the
mother hive cannot fpare it, *ib.*; and how to prevent a
late fwarm from coming off, 180; *see* Bees, Hives, and Re-
inforcing.

Swarming of bees, natural, preferable to artificial, when it can
be obtained, 149; the time uncertain, 150; attendance neceffary, *ib.*; variety of chances refpecting fwarming, *ib.*;
previous fymptoms, 151; a certain fign of its taking place,
ib.; manner of fwarming, *ib.*; 152; beautiful appearance in
the air. 152; noife unneceffary, except when the bees attempt
to fly off *ib.*; caution to be obferved, 153; means to make
them fettle, *ib.*; muft be carefully watched till the heat of the
day be over, 154; will fometimes fly off, notwithftanding
every method is ufed to prevent them, 155; young fwarms
fond of old hives, whofe bees are dead, 156; fuch hives often left on purpofe to entice them, by roguifh bee-mafters,
157; this equal to theft, *ib.*; and ought to be ftrictly
punifhed by law, *ib.*; a contrary decifion, however, *ib*;
criterion to determine, whether the hive was previoufly inhabited by living bees, 158; a fwarm will fly four miles to
a dead hive, *ib.*; they fly in a direct line, 159; directions
how to follow them, *ib.*; and fearch after them, *ib.*; 160;
161; decifive proof of their identity, 160; old trees,
churches, ruins, &c. fhould be fearched, 161; how to take
them out when difcovered, *ib.*; how to manage them
when the Queen cannot be got, 162; figns of a fecond or
third fwarming, *ib*; tolling, the young Queen's proclamation, or petition, defcribed, 163; very harmonious, 164;
an old Queen fometimes goes off with a colony, *ib.* 165;
two fwarms often join together, 166; method to prevent
this,

this, 167 ; if both fmall, rather advantageous, *ib.*, 168 ; various weights and numbers of fwarms, 168.

- **Swarms,** two, thrown annually in good years, 4 ; four taken off in one forenoon, 140 ; fometimes fly off, 155 ; two will often join together, 166 ; extraordinary number in one year, 225.

Sweat, on the ftool of a hive, defcribed, 151 ; when dried, a fymptom of an approaching fwarm, *ib.*

Syrup in the flowers, not changed, but extracted by the bees, 20, 22 ; different opinion urged by a correfpondent, 22 ; his experiment in proof of it, 23 ; *see* Honey.

T

Temper of the bees fhould be tried in artificial fwarming, 172.

Thorley, a writer on bees, 2 ; quoted, 164, 192 ; his account of the fmall white fcales carried in by the bees, 192 ; and the formation of wax, *ib.* ; 193 ; controverted, *ib.* 194, 195.

Tradefmen, country, advifed to keep bee-hives, 227 ; might have a hive for every hand they employ, *ib.*

Trees, fruit, of all kinds, the bloffoms of, afford honey, 15 ; benefit of planting, 40 ; *fee* Plane-trees.

Turnips, the flowers of, yield both honey and farina, 11 ; bloffom early, and continue long in flower, *ib.* ; fhould be fowed in fummer, 12 ; and allowed to run into flower in fpring, *ib.* ; advantage of rearing them, 40.

T

Uniting of bees, directions for, 135, *et seq.* ; *see* Hives, Re-inforcing, Swarming, &c.

V

Vices, bees have, as well as virtues, 116.

Villages, fome country, might have a hive for every houfe in them, 227.

Virgil

eather, good favourable to bees, 6, 7 ; bad, very hurtful to them, vii, 7, 8, 9, 29, 223 ; inconstancy of it, the only preventive of bees from thriving, 29 ; how to guard against its effects, vii. 223 ; *see* Cold, Heat, Rain, Wind, &c

eight of hives, that require supplies of food, 125, 126 ; of honey sufficient for that purpose, 126 ; of swarms, 168 ; of hives increased by changing their situations, 185 ; by the junction of swarms, 198 ; and by being long kept, *ib*

Theeler, George, Esq; his account of a repast of honey, 225, 226.

hite clover, white honey extracted from, 21.

hite matter thrown into the royal cells, by the bees, disquisition concerning it, 65, 66.

hite Stephen and W. writers on bees, 2 ; the former quoted, 103 ; and refuted, *ib*.

White thorn, honey dew observed on the leaves of, 19.

Wildman, Mr, a writer on bees, 2 ; quoted 19, 105 ; his reasoning upon the cold endured by bees in Russia, 105 ; controverted, *ib*. 106, 107, says that ants do not hurt bees, 222.

Wind hurtful to bees, 7, 29, 169.

Winter, how to prepare stock hives for, 95, 96, 97, 98 ; and to manage them in, 99, 100, 101, 102 ; a mild one supposed to be dangerous to bees, 103 ; this opinion refuted, *ib*. 104 : experiments, 107 ; severe winters sometimes kill whole hives, 197.

Wonders, seemingly incredible, which the author can perform with bees, 140, 141.

Wood lice hurtful to bees, 223 ; how to extirpate them, *ib*.

Wood, advantages of hives made of, 144

Working, or common bees, Schirach's opinion of, 54 ; any one capable, in an early stage, of becoming a Queen, *ib*. ; description of them, 78, 79, 80 ; differ in some particulars from both Queen and drones, 80, compose the whole community for three fourths of the year, 81 ; perform the whole labour of the hive, *ib*. ; and kill the drones, *ib*. ; unless hurt or affronted,

K k   fronted,

fronted, they seldom use their stings, 82; extremely irritable, *ib.*; directions how to handle them, *ib.*; their organs of smelling very acute, 84; they never sting when at work, 85; (*see* Sting;) not one of them should be killed, 200.

Worms, silk, analogous to bees, 196.

Y

Years peculiarly favourable to bees, viii. 4, 9, 105; probable increase of hives in ten, 5; ditto in seven, 47, 48; years hurtful to bees, 104.

Yellow, the fields and bees legs equally so, in May, 133.

Young bees sometimes found decayed in the cells, 128; (*see* Bees and Cells;) the more will be hatched, the longer the old ones remain in the hives, 202; how to preserve the young brood, when the honey is taken, *ib.,* 203.

Young swarms sometimes desert their hives, 123, *see* swarming.

Z

Zeal, patriotic, of the bees, in defence of their Queen and hive, 170, 171, *see* Queen, Wars, &c.

ADVERTISEMENT.

Any Gentleman, or Lady, who may be defirous of confulting or employing the Author of this work, with regard to the Management of Bees, in any refpect, upon addreffing a line to him at Mr GRANT'S, *Leith Wynd, Edinburgh, will be duely waited upon.*

The Author embraces this opportunity of returning his beft thanks to his numerous cuftomers in general, and to thofe of this metropolis in particular, for the very liberal encouragement he has repeatedly met with from them as a Honey Dealer; and begs that they will favour him with their orders, as early as poffible, for the honey of the enfuing feafon, to prevent danger of being difappointed.

EDINBURGH,
July 18. 1795.

ERRATA.

PAGE v Line 19th, For *both* read *all three.*
— 9 — 7th, For *does* read *do.*
— 21 — 21ft, For *connioffeurs* read *connoiffeurs.*
— 22 — 18th, For *meant* read *meat.*
— 22 — 27th, For *gentlemen* read *gentleman.*
— 27 — 26th, For *an article* read *articles.*
— 29 — 4th, For *preventative* read *preventive.*
— 31 — 21ft, and 22d, For *fhe prove a bad one and die,* read *moft or all of the bees die.*
— 37 — 16th, For *80,000,* read *320,000.*
— 47 — 29th, For *counties* read *countries.*
— 76 — 7th, For *breed* read *bred.*
— 120 — 19th, For *fome fore* read *a bloody.*
— 136 — 17th, For *her* read *it.*
— 149 — 2d, For *lon* read *lion.*
— — — 12th, For XIX read XX.
— 158 — 2d, For *no* read *every.*
— 159 — 13th, For *as* read *that.*
— — — 21ft, For *brufs* read *bufh.*
— 199 — 8th, For SWAMMERDANE read SWAMMERDAM.
— 210 — 3d, For *lever* read *fleeve.*
— 215 — 2d, For *flower,* read *flour.*
— — — 19th, For *fomented* read *fermented.*